MOVE

FOR

JOY

Cover design by Kim Li

Interior formatting by Dania Zafar

#MoveforJoybook

MOVE

FOR

JOY

AN INTUITIVE TRAINING APPROACH TO PURSUE GOD
IN FITNESS AND FIND HAPPINESS

KASEY SHULER

This book is dedicated to my clients: past, present, and future.

Download an Audiobook Sample for Free!

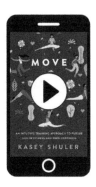

As a thank you for getting this book, I'd like to send you the first three chapters of Move for Joy on audiobook for free.

Go to www.kaseybshuler.com/moveforjoyaudio

Contents

ACT: WALK IT OUT   **157**

Introduction

You want the results of exercise: mirror-proof confidence, stress relief, increased energy, a sense of accomplishment, and longevity, but you don't want to actually *do* the exercise. Maybe you even have a fitness routine, but you either drag your feet or spend hours pumping iron and still feel deflated. Since fitness feels disconnected from your life and what you love, it comes and goes without any long-lasting consistency.

> *"Without exception... all try their hardest*
> *to reach the same goal, that is, joy."*[1]
> AUGUSTINE

We will do anything (even exercise when it's hard) for joy. The positive effects of fitness are temporary, but *Move for Joy* connects fitness with Jesus, the everlasting source of joy. Jesus is the One who holds all things together, and who can connect your fitness journey into mind, body, and soul health. This book will help you choose which of the five central motivators of fitness you relate to best. Each motivator, based on biblical and practical principles, will help you select exercises that release the positive physiological effects you need in the moment, while rooting your practice to a Joy Goal designed to flex with the changing seasons of your life.

    I've been in the fitness industry for ten years, but even longer if you count helping my mom in her at-home personal training studio, The Shape Shack (for those of you who have been looking for the perfect boutique gym name, you're welcome). In college, I earned a degree in health promotion and behavior because I am deeply interested not only in the *how* of health, but the *why*. In the health world, I know that we like food, and so we eat it. We don't like fitness, so we don't do it. I actually enjoyed fitness, but even I found myself loathing the idea of working out at times. How could I expect anything different from my personal training clients who struggled with over-eating and under-exercising? I started to ask myself the questions: Is it possible to like fitness as much as food? What if we could be filled up by reaching out? As I read Hebrews 12:2 about how Jesus endured the cross for the joy set before him, a light bulb turned on for me. Jesus was able to go to the cross to bring us joy. Maybe we could do the hard thing of exercise for the joy of being with Jesus.

In my initial assessments with coaching clients, I always ask, "What is your fitness goal?" It seems Tiffany was seeing the light too:

> *I am a professional bodybuilder who competed in figure competitions for two years. During that time, my life was completely 'me' focused. God has done a GREAT work in my life to reduce the grip I had on my body. It had become my idol. I restricted food and obsessed over everything I ate. I spent hours in the gym. Now that I'm not doing those things I often feel guilty. I know that guilt isn't from God. If I have an ice cream cone, I feel guilty and fat. If I don't work out, guilt. I've also gained weight. While I know it's probably healthy, I still feel guilty and like a failure. Back to those goals... Lately I've been thinking I need to set some fitness goals so I don't go to the other extreme of neglecting, or not honoring, my body. I struggle with setting goals because I don't want to be boxed in by them. I don't want it to seems as if I'm going back down that road of restriction. Does that make sense? As I'm typing this I can hear God saying, 'Come to me.' I must seek Him first. He'll help me strike the right balance.*

Like Tiffany, I knew many of my clients wanted more out of fitness than meets the eye, but didn't have the words to explain what they really needed. Their answers to the question, "What is your fitness goal?" began to settle into one of five categories. It turns out these categories are not only the five ways that modern fitness conglomerates hook consumers on the surface level, but each find its roots in the five ancient biblical purposes for the body. In my coaching services, I started connecting the answer to "What is my fitness goal?" to one of the five motivators. Immediately identifying with a core motivator helped my clients get to the heart of their fitness desires, to be filled with joy in the present, and fueled with joy for the journey ahead.

Female entrepreneurs, dads of toddlers, full-time teachers, digital nomads, and college students have all benefited from this focus on joy in their fitness practice. This is what these people said after a thirty-minute coaching call guiding them through the plan outlined in *Move for Joy*:

> *Your phone call was so incredibly helpful. Starting it and ending it with a prayer was wonderful. Just being able to talk through my issues and concerns with you was such a relief. I needed someone to remind me that I don't need to put so much pressure on myself, or hold myself to expectations that can't always be met. -Abby*

> *Blending the faith aspect was huge. -Rachel*

> *This call helped me sort out things in my brain and gave me accountability for my actions. You helped me progress my goal of walking to running with doable next steps. Thank you! -Lindsey*

> *It was nice to have someone to talk through this with and re-jumpstart my interest and focus on fitness. -Amanda*

It's been helpful because I see how God plays so much into this, and that's awesome. -Pamela

I've known how I feel and where I want to be, but having confirmation of how to get there is reassuring. Having you walk me through this helps me know I can do it. -Reina

It changes the why. If I'm overwhelmed with stuff, I think, 'this doesn't matter.' Reframing fitness and scheduling by what brings me peace reminds me fitness is important. It's the same overwhelm I've been experiencing with goal setting. I realize I like checking the boxes, but have a hard time coming up with goals. You helped me see that fitness facilitates the bigger goal. This method simplifies what you want to achieve so you can actually do it. -Danielle

I think you picked up this book because you want change. You want more than what every other fitness program is offering you. You want to know what exercises are right for you. You want to get to the heart of it all and walk away, breathlessly, ready for more!

Why does it feel so good to lie flat on the mat after a challenging workout? Because you put the right amount of work in and are experiencing the rewards of joy. If you sit down with this book (or read it on a recumbent bike), wrestle with the Lord through the hard questions, and put the plan into action, you will find joy.

Have you ever seen someone's face glowing? Maybe she was pregnant. Maybe he just worked out. Or maybe she just got a bright idea. In any case, the healthy glow comes from an inner flow, in which all parts feel integrated and work together to create and radiate joy. This is not an elusive phenomenon reserved for a select group of happy people. You too, can glow with joy. Jesus said, "Seek, and you will find." Seek Him, and you'll find joy. But be warned—this is not an easy road. You'll need to go through a bit of hardship on your journey. You will have Jesus as your companion and coach, and His joy will be your strength. He is always with you and will never leave you. Training joy will help your mind establish this truth.

I can't wait to hear what you will discover about the Lord, how He made you to move, and the impact that fitness can make on your Joy Goals. Nobody else can get fit for you. You get to take charge and make the next move. Which of the five motivators fits you? Which one defines your friends and family? Keep reading to find out!

ASSESS:
How Do You Feel
About Fitness?

CHAPTER ONE

When Working Out Isn't Working Out

"Sign up for the half marathon with me!" she said. "It will be fun!" she said. What she didn't know was that I had never run more than three miles in my life, and I couldn't understand why. Why run when you can drive? But it was 2008 and endurance events were trending in the fitness world, so I signed up to see what the hype was all about. All I could think was, "This race is going to be epic. And I'm going to feel so good about eating a lot of food afterwards." When reality set in and I sat down to inspect the training plan, my heart sunk: "I have to run *how much*?"

A race well beyond our ability requires training, the regular discipline of running...and running...and running some more. It all felt a little too time-consuming and way above my pay grade. But wait, I was the one paying for it. "How did my friend sucker me into this again?" I kept thinking as I pictured her bubbling over with excitement. Friendship will make you do crazy things. Even though my expectations were off and motivations misplaced, I learned a valuable lesson: training is the real race and joy is the finish line. I needed to find my joy.

Maybe you've bought into a fitness trend too, and walked away from it feeling like it wasn't your thing. If you've had a hard time figuring out what your "thing" is in fitness, I'm excited to share my journey with you. In the following chapters, you will discover the secret sauce of joy for our exercise endeavors, which of the five fitness motivators you identify with most, and learn how to create a movement plan that can stretch with every changing season of life.

Breaking Out of the Comfort Zone

Most of us simply struggle to get enough exercise to support our daily lives, let alone trying to train for marathons. To be exact, almost 30 percent of Americans[2] get no physical activity outside of normal tasks. About half of those who start an exercise program drop out within the first six months, and after two years, 80 percent have given up. These statistics have remained the same for thirty years.[3] It's not that this generation is lazy, but exercise is no longer convenient or even needed for most tech-heavy, developed countries.

Before the industrial revolution, people walked or rode bicycles to work and used their bodies for more tasks inside and outside of the house. To put it into perspective, studies have shown that Amish communities, which are comparable to past generations, spend about 40 percent of their day on manual labor.[4] Recreational and commercial fitness, as we know it today, is a mere 2 percent of our day (based on thirty minutes per day). Such a small amount of time spent on physical activity was simply unheard of until the 1950s.

If we took a look at the lives of adults in affluent places at any moment in the day, 70 percent would be sitting.[5] Not doing chores around the house or filling up water bottles or carrying kids... just... sitting. We sit for commutes. We sit to work on our laptops. We sit to eat. And, we sit to watch movies and read. I'm sitting on the floor right now to write this book!

Gyms refer to their members as athletes, because today, if you are in a gym, you are considered an athlete: one who *chooses* to go out of his or her way to exercise. Exercise is not the first way most people want to spend their time, not when there are cars with air conditioning to get us places quickly, phones to text your family member in the next room, and stimulating videos to watch in the palm of your hand, sterilely separated from the wild outdoors by a pane of glass.

Yo-Yo Exercising

Exercise, as communicated to us by fitness culture, can feel intimidating. We are supposed to buy expensive clothes and gym bags, remember to bring those clothes in said gym bag, take time out of our day, away from our families, to drive to the workout facility, do a workout we loathe to sweat enough to make it count, make time for a shower, and down a pricey organic protein shake. That's asking for hefty investments of time and money.

Then there are the degrading messages aimed at us through headlines and advertisement slogans:
- "Lose the Flab Fast" or "Earn the Body of Your Dreams" translate into: hurry up and change yourself because you aren't good enough as you are.
- "Burn Those Weekend Calories" insinuates that exercise is used as payment for poor nutrition choices, instead of a free gift.
- "Get Shredded in This Killer Workout" uses violent words to encourage us to tame our bodies, as if our bodies weren't an integral part of us.

These shameful metaphors only motivate us for a short time. When microwave meals became popular in the 1970s, healthy eating became hard, and diets were the temporary solution. Losing weight, repeatedly, by dieting and then gaining it back is called "yo-yo dieting." There's now the same term for exercising. I wonder if it's because we have bought into microwave fitness: do this one exercise and lose pounds in forty-five seconds!

And just as yo-yo dieting causes the body to hold onto even more fat, the result is the same for yo-yo exercising: "Sudden fitness regimens, rather like crash diets, appear to make our metabolism go into survival mode, responding to sudden bouts of sustained exertion by trying its best to preserve energy."[6] We need to become aware of what we need, find a style of fitness appropriate for our season of life, and continue to adapt as long as we both shall live. Sound like a marriage proposal? We get one body to have and love for the rest of our lives, so let's make this an enjoyable relationship!

Take a look at the top six reasons people don't work out[7]:

1. I don't have time.
2. I'm too tired.
3. I don't get a break from the kids.
4. Exercise is boring.
5. I don't like to move.
6. I've tried it before.

To quickly debunk the above, each of us can honestly admit that there's time in the world for anything worthwhile. Exercise gives you more energy when you're tired. You can work out with your kids. You can find something fun that fits with your lifestyle. I realize I sound like a typical personal trainer, making exercise easier than it sounds, without acknowledging the very real curve balls of life. But, there is truth here that helps us see the reasons for what they are: excuses that can be overcome. It's not that we can't exercise or that moving is too hard, it's just that deep down, we don't want to get out of our comfort zones.

Because as William James, philosopher and psychologist noted, "How to gain, how to keep, how to recover happiness, is in fact for most men at all times the secret motive of all they do, and of all they are willing to endure." The goal of this book is to strengthen the presence of joy, and in turn, weaken the power of pain. The more we associate fitness with joy, the more we will pursue it.

Before we start with the dictionary definition, how would you personally define fitness?

_____

_____

_____

Who, what, or which life experiences fed your definition?

_____

_____

_____

On the scale below, mark where you would categorize yourself from couch potato to fit as a fiddle:

On the same scale above, mark, with a star, where you would like to be.

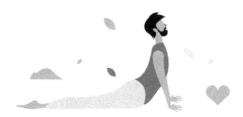

Here are three definitions of fitness:
1. Health
2. Capability of the body to distribute inhaled oxygen to muscle tissue during increased physical effort
3. Also called **Darwinian fitness**. *Biology.*
   a. the genetic contribution of an individual to the next generation's gene pool relative to the average for the population, usually measured by the number of off-spring or close kin that survive to reproductive age.
   b. the ability of a population to maintain or increase its numbers in succeeding generations.[8]

Why Do We Need To Be Fit?

If we combine all of the above definitions, the basic role of fitness in our lives is the ability to adapt to varying conditions and reproduce. Living in the age of technology, our conditions change too rapidly for the human body to keep up. We are tempted to outpace technology, but if we do, we will become as fragmented as the machines we depend on. Our goal as human beings is holistic strength, to be ready and willing to change with the seasons. The mind-body connection, the integration of joy, is key to adaptation.

The real measure of fitness is our ability to experience a stressful situation and bounce back quickly. How strong is our home base, and how quickly can we return home again? Instead of being able to beat the clock on a run, experts now look at vagal tone (the activity of the nerve connecting the gut and brain) as measured by heart rate variability. After being exposed to a high-intensity sprint, how quickly does the heart rate return to resting and continue delivering oxygen at a steady pace?

A restful state is also crucial to reproduction. A woman at peace feels abundantly safe to release nourishment to grow another life, but stress sends the body into survival mode and hoards vital resources. A good takeaway is not to be stressed about having a visible six-pack. Neither stress nor having min-iscule amounts of body fat are actually beneficial to the fitness of the human race.

Exercise is the training ground for all-around life fitness. Training the body in a controlled setting makes us feel the joy of being connected within, which allows us to rest and bring forth life, both in ourselves and for others. If fitness is adaptation and reproduction, then by the end of this book you will know not only how to adapt *to* your life conditions, but adapt life *for* your Joy Goal.

Besides doing the obvious, like keeping your weight in check, empowering you to lift heavy things, decreasing anxiety and depression, and reducing your risk for a host of other diseases, here are three benefits of exercise that could come as a surprise:

1. **Exercise makes you smarter** (decreases depression, increases memory recall and focus, shown to help prevent Alzheimer's) by increasing blood flow to the brain to feed blood vessels and create new brain cells.[9]

2. Contrary to popular belief that sweating causes skin breakouts, sweat opens the pores and lets out all the toxins, which acts as a natural (and cheap) detoxifier[10] and **improves skin quality**.

3. Except for those times when you're blasting music through your headphones, **exercise enhances your hearing skills** by improving blood flow to the inner ear, and preventing the loss of neurotransmitters, which carry the signals to your brain,[11] allowing you to detect robberies in action across the city so you can fly to the rescue… or simply to hear your name being called across a busy Starbucks.

How Much Exercise Do I Need?

If you don't like exercise but want the benefits, you may be won-dering, how much should I exercise? All the time! Before I lose you, let me explain. Many circuit training workouts have led us to believe that we need to exercise for at least thirty minutes for it to count. While twenty minutes of sustained activity does improve the cardiovascular system, sometimes we only have ten minutes of uninterrupted time to move at a fast pace, and that's okay too.

Katy Bowman, in her book *Move Your DNA,* puts exercise under the umbrella of movement, which is going on all day long (even in your sleep as you roll around). She compares movement with eating, a habit we take joy in doing, and encourages her readers to engage in nutritious movement: "Nutritious Movement is a whole-body movement program that utilizes exercises, alignment adjustments, and habitat (lifestyle) changes to better move all trillion of your body's parts."[12] Think of moving your body all day as your meal, and a scheduled exercise session as your supplement. A supplement is secondary to a nutrient-dense meal and catered to your individual needs.

Instead of thinking of exercise as a separate activity to fit in a few times a week, consider how you can move more throughout your day, whether that be parking far away, ditching the technology in favor of manual chores, or even something seemingly insignificant, like going barefoot (in safe places) to make better use your feet and ankle joints. Ultimately, how much exercise you need depends on your Joy Goal, which we will define in the next chapter. If we can discover what brings us joy and connect exercise with the very fabric of our core desires, exercise no longer becomes a separate task. Movement will grow as a natural extension of ourselves.

What Happens If I Don't Exercise?

Here's where we get into the cost-benefit analysis of movement. Sitting is "the new smoking"[13] simply because the body is inactive. Standing could be the new smoking if all you did was stand in one place. Being sedentary most of the day strongly increases the risk for cardiovascular disease, type 2 diabetes, colon, and lung cancer.[14] These consequences are all disease-oriented, but we can't discount the effects our sedentary lifestyle has on the next generation's mental health.

In a study that measured sedentary screen time over two to three hours per day in adolescents, scientists discovered strong associations with "depressive symptomatology. Other mental health measures were: anxiety symptoms, self-esteem, suicide ideation, loneliness, stress, and psychological distress."[15] According to the World Health Organization, depression is the leading cause of disability in the US and Canada, ranking above coronary heart disease, cancer, and AIDS.[16] When we busy our minds without moving our bodies, our whole selves suffer. Depression is a type of hibernation, but exercise pulls us out of the mental cave and into the light, one step at a time. Exercise is like the body's outreach ministry. One study shows that every fifty minutes of weekly exercise reduces the risk of depression by 50 percent, and that a regular vigorous exercise routine is just as effective as anti-depression medication. To put a spin on Newton's first law of motion, a person at rest unravels into unrest, but a person in motion releases positive emotions. Exercise is medicine, and joy is the spoonful of sugar.

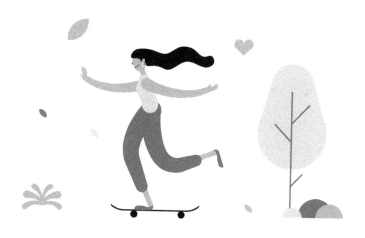

In the chart below, fill in the boxes with how exercise makes you feel when you do it (or have done it in the past) and the consequences of not exercising.

Type of exercise	How I feel afterward	How I feel skipping exercise

Referring to the filled in chart above, is exercise worth the effort?

_____

_____

_____

What's Your Shark Slide?

Our four-year-old friend's birthday party was on a hot summer day in Georgia, and as the adults lounged on picnic tables in the shade, munching on leftover pimento cheese and chicken salad, the kids ran around screaming, digging mud holes, and tumbling down a shark water slide. Some of the parents remarked on how much fun it looked like they were having. The host of the party said, "Next time, we can rent one for the adults too!" We nodded our heads like it was a fantastic idea. I was pregnant at the time, and as I smiled in masked agreement, I laughed to myself, "No way, mister," and then with a pretense of pessimism, "Even if I weren't pregnant, that would never happen. Preschool parent acquaintances getting in their bathing suits and sliding down an inflatable water slide with all the internal body judgement and slide performance evaluations? Eh… " I dismissed the thought as clearly unrealistic, and definitely not joyful.

A shark water slide is enough motivation for kids to get active, but what about adults? We are the ones who are supposed to be setting healthy examples. But clearly, I built up too many insecurities to race down an inflatable water slide with other parents. If that's true, then what motivates adults to move? What is *our* shark slide? If we can find a reason to get excited about working out, that highly-charged emotional energy will not only lead us to move, but the energy of a workout will feed excitement for the future and establish positive memories for more.

The Truth in Fitness Marketing

While marketing ploys can use negative fitness metaphors and perpetuate unattainable expectations, we can learn valuable lessons from marketing research. The marketing model works to understand the needs of customers and business practices, which then develops ways to fulfill those needs and, in effect, make money to keep doing more of what works and studies what does not. As a personal trainer with a background in health promotion and behavior, I too want to know what people need to help them succeed. Instead of using the stick approach and bringing out a bullhorn and drill sergeant whistle to change external behaviors, I piggybacked off fitness advertising to find the donuts (or carrots) of internal motivation. I scoured magazines and blog headlines and discovered that every line of advertising fit into one of five needs, and they lined up with the reasons people joined a gym in 2016[17]:

1. Thirty-eight percent of people joined a gym to get a better looking body. This correlates with **the need to feel confident in one's body** and aligns with these headlines: "Hot and Happy," "Fit at Any Size," or "Strong and Sexy."
2. Thirty-nine percent go to the gym to provide counterbalance to stress in everyday life, which is **the need to relieve stress**. The messages of "Instant Calm," or "Anxiety and Your Heart" connect with this need.
3. Forty-one percent joined a gym to lose weight, which fits with **the need to be more productive**: "24 Wellness Hacks," "Instant Energy Upgrade," or "Energy Blast" would fit this market.
4. Forty-one percent joined a gym to optimize strength and endurance, and twenty-five percent to meet friends. This desire is **the need to win at life**. The health magazines would say something like: "Think You Can Handle This Circuit?", "500 KG Squat," or "Crossfit's Toughest Workout."
5. Fifty-four percent joined a gym to be healthy, fulfilling **the need to take care of oneself**. This self-care desire lines up with the following: "Rewind Skin Damage," "Nourish Your Body," or "10 Ways to Injury-Proof Your Body."

Becoming media literate wakes us up to the messages we unconsciously absorb. It helps us ask ourselves, "What are they selling, and why do I want to buy it?" The average American currently spends $155 per month on health and fitness, as outlined below, which equates to $112,000 over a lifetime. As a disclaimer, this survey was conducted by a protein company, so it's no surprise that they made this study public, as supplements are first on the list. The wise person would invest in a trusted personal trainer, who can provide advice for the rest of the health and fitness purchases.* Here's the breakdown of our spending, according to their findings:

- 36% supplements
- 22% gym clothing
- 22% gym memberships
- 11% meal plans or nutritional advice
- 9% personal trainer[18]

DISCLAIMER: This message is funded by a personal trainer.

Assess your Situation

How much money per month do you spend on:

Supplements	
Gym clothing	
Gym memberships	
Meal plans or nutritional advice	
Personal training	

Over 2,000 years ago, Jesus spoke truthfully when He said, "For where your treasure is, there your heart will be also" (Matthew 6:21). The focus of marketing is to determine the desires of our hearts, and our wallets will follow, and vice versa.

What do your investments in fitness say about your heart?

_____

_____

_____

In what ways has investing in fitness shaped your heart?

_____

_____

_____

Over 90 percent of our purchasing decisions are subconscious.[19] That means most of our decisions are based on intuition, or feeling. When my friend Erin shared her story with me about why she started exercising and how she has stuck with it, I heard a lot of emotional words, which I've emphasized for you.

> *I have finally found an exercise **that I love**. With running I would get obsessed with how fast I was going and how many calories I was burning. And then my left knee started bothering me pretty bad. I decided to do a trial month of*

*hot yoga. I had already done it before, but becoming a member of a studio seemed financially impossible. After the trial month my husband noticed a huge difference in my confidence and said that we needed to do whatever we could to keep it in my life because of how much **happier** I was. He was so right. It has been a game changer for me. When I go to class, I notice improvement, without worrying about numbers. I used to approach the gym with anxiety, but this class has taught me how incredibly the same we all are. Ultimately, **I exercise to feel better**. It used to be so that I would look better. But after years of torturing myself with that mindset, I realized that for me, how I feel is the most important thing. When I leave a hot yoga class I feel healthy, motivated, accomplished, and beautiful.*

Can I say that I **love** her story? Her exercise journey began with a superficial focus on proving herself, but what actually transformed her was focusing on her most important thing.

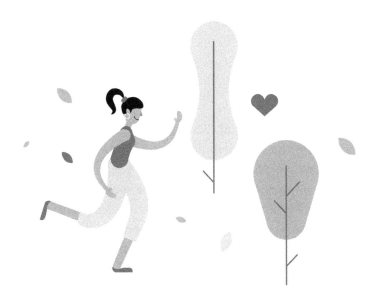

What is your most important thing? How do you want to feel today? How about tomorrow?

_____

_____

_____

_____

_____

Exercise is a means to joy. It can give us immediate gratification, which feels good and makes us want more. But since the happy feelings will evaporate with the sweat, you need a long-term plan. In Chapter Two, we will lay out a seasonal Joy Goal for you, and get you started on one of five paths of:
1. Confidence
2. Peace
3. Effectiveness
4. Victory
5. Health

As Charles Spurgeon said, "As there is the most heat nearest to the sun, so is the most happiness nearest to Christ." To make your joy last, we will hitch that fitness wagon to a star—and connect your journey with the Lord, the source of light and joy. Then we will plan practical next steps towards your Joy Goal by incorporating the discipline you need and discovering the way God designed you, putting up bumpers along the path to keep you on track.

How exactly do we connect fitness with Jesus? I was

pleasantly surprised to find that in my search of digging into the five surface-level reasons for exercising, I found they correlated with five of the Bible's core purposes for our body.

Marketing Messages	Our Needs, Filled in Christ	Biblical Proof
Feel confident	Look to Jesus for *confidence*	Body is a covering of glory (Col. 3:12)
Relieve stress	Meet with Jesus for *peace*	Body is a temple (1 Corin. 6:19)
Energize	Be filled with Jesus for Kingdom *effectiveness*	Body is a vessel (2 Tim. 2:21)
Win at life	Join with Jesus's body for *victory*	Body is a member of the body (Ephesians 4:15-16)
Be healthy	Listen to Jesus to create a *healthy* body	Body is a home (2 Corin. 5:9)

God gave us these desires for a reason. Like a girl trying to make it to the finish line, or a shark slide to a kid, these motivators were handed to us not as a final stop, but something to follow. The motivators are on the outside to draw us in to the center. The center is the goal, and we need to know what our goal is if we want to get there: "[Setting goals] is merely setting a direction for your life. You are going to go somewhere so how much better to have a direction that has been set by communion with the divine Center."[20]

Many people discontinue their pursuit in the same direction once they get superficial results. But please, don't stop there! You won't be fully satisfied and will keep searching for something more. As A.W. Tozer observed, "Man is bored, because he is too big to be happy with that which sin is giving him."[21] This short-term goal is a false finish line—the lost weight and improved energy are simply gifts that can only be truly enjoyed when we connect them to the Gift-Giver.

We must battle the temptation for worldly comfort, whether that's something as harmless as an easy chair or the looming fear of trying again and failing. If you've ever tried to get up early to work out, you know that taking care of yourself is a battle. And the stakes are high!

Satan wants to kill, steal, and destroy. He will destroy you through the subtle means of slowly killing the body by discouraging and distracting the spirit. If you feel resistance in your exercise efforts, it might be because you are valuable and your vigor is a threat to the dominion of darkness. Let us stay alert, awake, and on top of his schemes. Get behind us, Satan. We're moving forward in joy, for joy!

Make a Victory Circle

As you may have discovered in other successful endeavors, the road to freedom is not a straight path. And sometimes, God leads us around the very thing that threatens us to display His omnipotence, like a bird circling its prey. Remember the walls of Jericho. God did not lead the Israelites straight through the city with shows of force, but around the walls of their enemy, seven times, with shouts of praise. Beforehand, the Lord told Gideon, [Joshua?] "I *have* given Jericho into your hand."[22] Notice the emphasized past-tense word in that verse. Jericho was the one obstacle standing in the way of the Israelites and the Promised Land. On the seventh lap, God's people let out a shout of victory *before* the walls came down.

The Lord might lead you right back to where you started, to the very class or program or people that made you feel inadequate, to show you that He has already won. Like the people marching around Jericho, like one person jogging around a track, like all of humanity hurtling back to utopia, you might find that when you get back to the start, you are at the finish.

My half-marathon was the perfect example. The only way I made it through the race that day was prayer. When I thought I was almost there, but looked up in utter despair at the flag overhead reading, "Mile Six," I almost gave up right then and there. But before I could make up my mind, it was like an angel swooped in and started carrying me on by prayer: "I can do all things in Christ…" I repeated with each step until my last. I heard the roar from the crowds gathered on the sidelines, like the great cloud of witnesses. As I flew across the finish line of the half-marathon with arms wide open, I imagined receiving the prize of Jesus' words: "Well done, good and faithful servant… enter into the joy of your master" (Matthew 25:23).

Walls of Jericho Exercise

Which of the six reasons for not exercising resonate with you? Circle all that apply.

1. I don't have time.
2. I'm too tired.
3. I don't get a break from the kids.
4. Exercise is boring.
5. I just don't like to move.
6. I've tried it before.

"Measure the size of the obstacles against the size of God."
BETH MOORE

Just as you circled the words above, circle your obstacle with your feet. You can practice at home by putting the object that represents your struggle on the ground (like a planner to represent "I don't have time") and walking around it in a wide circle. Every time you make one revolution, say, "The Lord has given [insert obstacle] into my hand." On the seventh time around, declare victory by raising your arms in praise, and giving a big shout, knowing that God fights your battles as you joyfully walk in faith. This exercise may feel strange to do, but it is so powerful. Try it and see for yourself!

CHAPTER TWO

Training Joy

"This looks like a good hike—it's only three miles and the description mentions breathtaking views at the top!" I shared excitedly with my husband, not knowing how to actually navigate a trail. The only other long hikes in unknown places I had attempted was with my expert, REI-employed friend, but I figured I knew enough from those experiences to give it a go. He shrugged in agreement and drove us to the trailhead. We found it and started our adventure. He moved aside fallen tree branches while I recited facts about all the physical benefits of this hike. After I ran out of interesting tidbits, and it felt like we had been walking for way longer than one-and-a-half miles, he voiced my suspicions and asked, "Are you sure this was a loop trail?" I tried to hide my look of certain uncertainty.

I'm not the best with directions. I use Google Maps everywhere, and would have used it if we had cell service in the middle of the woods. Eventually, we ran into a lone hiker (our guardian angel) and he confirmed that we were, in fact, going the right way, and that an amazing view was just up ahead. When there was no more incline, the trees opened up to a spectacular panorama of mountains and open air. Phew! I didn't completely fail us.

The view was breathtaking, but experiencing it with my husband was what made it so wonderful. What I learned was that joy is not just the achievement at the top, but walking the path together. Together, being the key word. As we hiked, talked, nearly got lost, bonded over my less-than-expert navigation skills, and shared an amazing vista side by side, I felt together on the inside too. It was one of those times when I realized how joy is not just an endpoint, but experiencing the journey with all its ups and downs. When we move our bodies, we experience a full integration of our feelings, our thoughts, and our actions: an all-encompassing sensation of joy. It's a feeling that overflows and naturally wants to reach out to share. When we invite the Lord on our journey, He connects all the pieces in the joy circuit, and becomes a fire in our heart and a lamp to our feet.

The Immediate Rewards of Exercise

This feeling is not just for fun. Joy is built into our design for survival. All the essentials of living, and keeping humanity alive for generations, bring us similar abundant pleasure: eating, sleeping, moving, reproducing, and helping one another out all produce joy. In *Wired for Joy*, the author explains how each decision we make elicits feelings of stress or joy, like two paths diverging in a wood. Sharing, cooperating, and doing society good elicits positive feelings of joy (eudonic rewards), which ensures the survival of humanity as a whole. This is the long-term solution. Community-centered evolutionary response is countered by stress, which is an individual-focused survival response (fueled by hedonistic rewards), the short-term escape solution. Joy turns us to help each other and keeps us balanced, and stress turns us inward to help ourselves and keep us alive.

While stress is a very useful response when we are in imme-diate and real danger, it seems to creep into our lives far more often than necessary, overloading our systems, and is the cause of almost 95 percent of all health maladies. If we make too many stress-oriented decisions, we build up an "allostatic load" of stress, accumulating the resulting toxic neurochemicals within us, making us feel stressed-out instead of blissed-in.

While these neurochemicals have their place, flooding the

brain with an excessive amount of the following can result in unpleasant symptoms:

- **Adrenaline:** Too much adrenaline will leave you feeling jittery and unable to focus on priorities. If levels do not subside, adrenaline can keep heart rate and blood pressure elevated.
- **Cortisol** in copious amounts can give you an upset stomach, alters the immune system, suppresses the digestive system, the reproductive system, and other growth processes. An overload of cortisol initiates gluconeogenesis, which breaks down protein from muscle into glucose and is stored as fat if unused.

When we are constantly in survival mode, or fight-or-flight mode, we can suffer long-term effects like anxiety, depression, digestive problems, headaches, sleep disorders, weight gain, memory and concentration impairment, and even heart disease.

Stress as a necessary tool, but joy is our home. When we make a decision that leads to joy and re-establishes homeostasis, we feel empowered, balanced, confident, energized, and filled with good pleasure. Recreational drugs narrow the receptors and produce fewer chemicals with each use, so the user builds up a tolerance and constantly needs more. But exercise expands the receptors to receive more happy neurochemicals:

- **Endocannabinoids** released with exercise make us feel euphoric, content, and mellow.
- When we set a goal and achieve it, we release **dopamine**, making us feel more extroverted.
- Face-to-face contact with others releases **oxytocin**, the bonding chemical that increases trust and loyalty.
- Physical exertion releases **endorphins**, our body's natural morphine, making us more resistant to pain.
- **GABA** (the anti-anxiety molecule) creates calm by slowing down neuron activity. Release this by doing mindful activities.

- Pursuing meaningful challenges releases **serotonin**, the confidence molecule, which increases levels of worthiness and self-esteem.
- **Adrenaline** is the energy chemical that makes you feel a rush of life, and is released when you step outside your comfort zone and take a risk. [23]

Endorphin-induced feelings of runner's high and the dopamine-powered confidence are wonderful all on their own, but they serve a greater purpose. While happiness is based on what happens, joy is deeper and longer-lasting. These good feelings are designed not only to help us survive in this world, but to lead us to the God of eternal joy. Below, Amanda shares how Jesus is transforming her fitness goals for joy:

I'm a reformed fitness and wellness lover. Fitness used to be a box to check, in my life of things I had to do, to pursue the ideal 'me.' It was coupled with a crippled understanding of my identity and a desire to control my own life. Cue years of feeling less-than, not enough, too much and too little simultaneously—too many subtle lies whispered to my heart that sounded a lot like devastating truths. I overate and starved myself in pursuit of appeasing the ever-elusive lies, which were never satisfied.

Then Jesus comes in and shatters it all to rebuild this idea of wellness of body, mind, and soul rooted and grounded in Him. Step-by-step, inch by inch, Jesus is redeeming this whole idea of wellness in my life. It's been decades in the making. His work is never slow. It is always on time. And don't you know that He delights in doing this little by little work in us? It's for His glory, for our joy, and for the good of those around us.

Just as the rewards of happy feelings await us through physical movement, so the rewards of faith await us by drawing near to

God: "And without faith it is impossible to please him, for whoever would *draw near* to God must believe that he exists and that he rewards those who seek him" (Hebrews 11:6, emphasis added). Faith lies not just in believing that God exists (even the demons believe in Jesus, and tremble), but believing that God is good and rewards (not punishes or condemns) those who move toward Him with whole heart, soul, and strength.

If you can picture God's face toward you, what is His expression? Does your view make you want to draw near or back off?

_____

_____

_____

What experiences informed that picture, and do you think those are an accurate reflection of Him?

_____

_____

_____

Do you believe that He wants to reward you? If so, how?

_____

_____

_____

Laying the Foundation: Jesus Pursued You for the Joy

If you struggle to move toward God, remember how He always takes the first step:

> "And the angel said to them, 'Fear not, for behold, I bring
> you good news of great joy that will be for all the people.
> For unto you is born this day in the city of David a Savior,
> who is Christ the Lord. And this will be a sign for you: you
> will find a baby wrapped in swaddling cloths and lying in
> a manger'" (Luke 2:10-12).

The word "joy" was used plenty of times in the Old Testament. But when Jesus entered the world in the New Testament, the writers of the Bible described joy as "grace recognized." God's people had been waiting and working for thousands of years for God's promises to come to fruition. And finally, what they had been waiting for, *grace*, the forgiveness of sins through Christ, was here! They were filled with the gladness of grace. Joy is ful-*fill*-ment.

The angel gave them a physical sign to follow and receive their joy. But not all came to worship the baby Jesus. The scribes who told the wise men where the King was to be born in Bethlehem knew exactly where He was, but didn't go and see Him. They may have known the source of joy in their heads, but their feet didn't move in response. They missed out on real joy!

The Bible often describes seeking the Lord with action words. Highlight the verbs in the verses below:

- "Come to me, all who are weary and heavy laden, and I will give you rest." Matthew 11:28
- "Was no one found to return and give praise to God except this foreigner?' And he said to him, 'Rise and go your way; your faith has made you well.'" Luke 17:19
- "And he arose and came to his father. But while he was still a long way off, his father saw him and felt compassion, and ran and embraced him and kissed him." Luke 15:20

On our way to Jesus, he rewards us with the peace of rest. On our way back from praising Jesus, He fills us up to pour His joy out to others. And as we return to him like the prodigal son, no matter how many times, He *runs* to us. Can you imagine how His face lights up when He sees us turning to Him?

Messages of fitness culture include individual effort, no excuses allowed, and a bit of shame is necessary for proper motivation. No, my friends, not in the Lord. There is no condemnation on His face. Whether you have never worked out a day in your life, or have exercised for all the wrong reasons, Jesus keeps no record of wrongs. He came down from heaven for you, went to the cross for you, and is with you!

> *"Who for the joy that was set before him endured the cross, despising the shame, and is seated at the right hand of the throne of God" (Hebrews 12:2).*

As your face was the joy for Him set beyond the cross, so is His face the joy set before us on our fitness journey *and* beyond the pain of perseverance. We are free to experience the joy of salvation not as a one-time event, but a lifelong journey with Him. This is the difference between a simple runner's high and running with the Lord Most High: a runner's high fades like a battery-powered lamp, while the joy of the Lord is an energy source we have constant connection to. Moving our feet in faith flips the joy switch, and His presence sustains us throughout life— this life and the next!

Joy is a Unified Circuit

There are three areas of brain function:
1. **Architectural:** Three parts working together
2. **Electrical:** Neurological paths of thought
3. **Chemical:** Neurochemical rewards

We have a triune brain, a trinitarian picture of how three separate parts work together for one purpose, and when all parts
work together, we feel the wholeness of joy. It's amazing how we
are made in His image! While all parts are equally important,
there is a hierarchy of authority. The lower reptilian brain con-
tains our instincts, the middle limbic brain houses our emotions,
and the upper neocortex is the watchtower of high order
thinking.

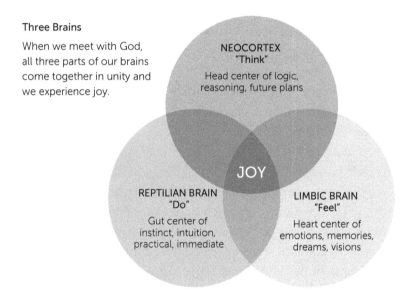

Three Brains

When we meet with God,
all three parts of our brains
come together in unity and
we experience joy.

NEOCORTEX
"Think"

Head center of logic,
reasoning, future plans

JOY

REPTILIAN BRAIN
"Do"

Gut center of
instinct, intuition,
practical, immediate

LIMBIC BRAIN
"Feel"

Heart center of
emotions, memories,
dreams, visions

While the upper brain gives executive orders, it's not always the
one in charge. Interestingly, there is no central command center
in the brain. Whichever area gets the most stimulation is the
one that leads. For example, when we are plagued with stress,
the lower reptilian brain takes over and we live out of survival
mode. We need a King for our competitive brain. Scripture says
that "in Him, all things hold together" (Colossians 1:17, NIV).
Our joy is found not by leaning on our own understanding and
forcing rational thoughts, but letting the cross be the connection
between the synapses.

In addition to an integrated brain, the mind-body relationship is crucial to joy. Our brain tells our body to move, and our body gives our brain information through kinesthetic receptors found in muscles, joints, and tendons. This mutual exchange keeps us in tune with our internal and external environment, but the order in which we make decisions is not always clear. I know that whenever I am anxious, the Lord begins to center me by bringing internal awareness of my fixed spot in space. One specific cue He gave me was, "Look at your feet." When I did, I was reminded that I was not actually dwelling in an anxious unknown future, but I was present and grounded in my body. My thoughts felt pulled together in peace. Our brain may direct much of our behavior, but our body is essential to understanding our basic needs and anchoring us to reality, which may get lost in the vortex of thought life. Neither is more important than the other, only the connection between the two.

We all have mind-body imbalances caused by mini traumas, whether that's insecurity over not being athletic or fit enough, or the fear of getting injured again, so let's begin closing the joy circuit by using a bottom-up approach and relearn how to be in our bodies. First, we **assess** our input (feel), then **ask** new questions (think), and finally, **act** (do). Once we are okay with feeling our feelings and tuning in to our somatic signals, our upper brain can resume making rational choices according to our assessed needs. Exercise itself is both a bottom-up and top-down activity: movement nudges the brain stem to produce the energy and interest to move, while the neocortex releases the reward neurochemicals like serotonin and endorphins to keep us going. Now that you have an idea of why this all works, let's get to work on laying out our joy journey path.

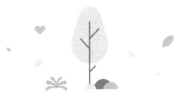

ASSESS (Feel)

What Do I Not Need?

I was not a regular hiker, but I had learned from experience with my REI-employed, expert adventurer friend that to reach the amazing views, the first step was to find the trailhead. Sometimes, the most obvious trailhead to body awareness is pain. We are usually moved to exercise because we are lacking in some area: we feel stressed and need to get out for some fresh air; a trip up the stairs that leaves us out of breath leads us to get on the treadmill; we are feeling "fat" (like the extra skin coming out of our waistband, life feels chaotic and out of our control), and need to take action. Perhaps the most painful scenario is not a visceral feeling, but a projected scenario like failing to reach or set life goals. Pain-based motivation is not what we are looking for, but it can be used to point to pleasure. Let us gently uncover the pain to find the source of our healing.

Like a patient at a doctor's office, you picked up this book because you have a pain point with fitness. What's not working out for you?

_____

_____

_____

_____

_____

Most of our memories and subconscious feelings are stored in the middle brain, the limbic brain. Every emotion has a memory tied to it. If you feel down and consider going to the gym but feel like you don't belong, it could be from that time when someone side-eyed you because didn't know how to use the machines. If you think about signing up for a neighborhood kickball league because you need social interaction, but exercise gives you anxiety, that feeling may be attached to the memory of when you were constantly called out by the coach growing up. If you want to do something adventurous but see exercise as frivolous and feel guilty for indulging, it might be from that time you signed up for a race and your husband said it was a waste of money. If you're feeling like you're not yourself and want to uncover your potential by losing extra pounds but feel shameful about exercise, maybe it's from that awful memory of the middle school boy saying something about your size at recess.

If you have negative feelings about exercise, what memory could it be attached to?

_____

_____

_____

_____

_____

Below is a visual of the Hebbian learning theory: "neurons that fire together, wire together." When you see a banana, and the neurons responsible for recognizing certain characteristics like, "yellow," "curved," and "smooth" fire together consistently, they start building synaptic bridges toward one another, and over time, make an associative group your brain recognizes as a "banana."

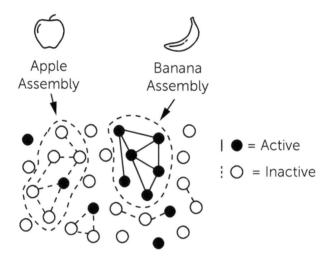

This learning model illustrates why you might currently associate the word "fitness" with "dread." What I don't want you to do is keep doing things that you don't like, or that do not help, and continue to activate those neurons to fire together and associate fitness as a pain to be avoided at all costs. For example, if you dislike sweat, pain, and spandex, yet these three things are consistently associated with your fitness experience devoid of positive feelings, your memory of fitness will be of that terrible trio.

Feelings of guilt and shame that ignite the stress response are stored in your memories, and likewise stored in the neuromuscular junctions associated with your memory. Just as dogs shake vigorously after an episode of aggression or to shake off excess water, we can use movement to shake out the unwanted feelings that lodge within us. One of the best ways to get the whole body shaking is through laughter. Even fake laughter gets the ball rolling! Try it out with a friend and see if this little challenge doesn't end in some real belly laughs.

Getting to express our emotion through motion is healthy. And in fact, *not* expressing emotion can lead to unwanted stress buildup, even disease, according to the first stage of the six stages of disease in Ayurvedic principles[24]:

1. Accumulation
2. Aggravation
3. Transmigration
4. Localization
5. Manifestation
6. Complication

The first step of disease is accumulation. Often, we have too much of one thing (the same repetitive movements, extra calories, etc.) and the harmful effects have to overflow somewhere. Let's stop for a minute and pinpoint what we do not need, to open up room to receive what we do need. This may be one of the most important parts of exercising: meeting that temptation face-to-face and getting to say what it is no longer welcome. Your body needs protection from excess, and you are her first defense! I say "her," because despite how culture objectifies the body, your body is not an "it," but a "she" or "he"—your body is *you*! When you treat your body as a person, you will love her, appreciate her, and treat her as a person.

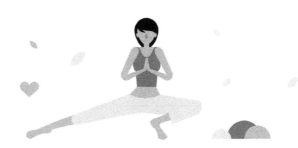

Write a thank you letter to your body, and then say what she or he does not need, as if you were speaking to the most intimate of friends. Remember to use gendered pronouns: her or him.

_____

_____

_____

_____

_____

_____

_____

_____

_____

_____

_____

_____

_____

_____

_____

_____

Get it out

One particular study shows how crying emotional tears releases stress hormones, and any other accumulated toxins from stress. Crying can also stimulate the production of endorphins.[25]

Release the fear

A natural reaction to fear is to draw the knees in and curl up into a fetal position of comfort and familiarity. Since the hips are used to draw in the knees, they can become tense when the mind is constantly riddled by fear. Try and settle into this Child's Pose hip opener for 12 breaths.

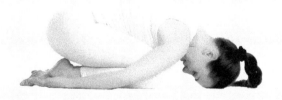

Release the guilt and shame

Guilt and shame make you feel like you want to hide from the world, so the body instinctively collapses at the chest, slumping the shoulders and head forward and down, which also increases neck pain. Take a step in releasing guilt and shame by doing Camel Pose for 3-6 breaths, or until you feel the tension of surrendering your mind and lifting your heart.

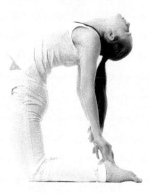

Release the anxiety

When it feels like we are holding the weight of the world on our shoulders, we tend to lift them up to support the mental weight, which also restricts the movement of our diaphragm and makes our breathing shallow, perpetuating the feeling of not being able to catch one's breath. Release the anxiety and tension in your shoulders by trying Rag Doll, allowing your knees to bend and letting your arms hang or gently sway in loose circles until you feel at ease.

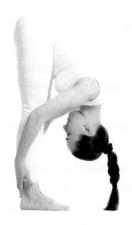

ASK (Think)

What Is Your Joy Goal?

We are motivated by immediate gratification because we exist in the present. We are moved by thinking, "I'm tired and need energy," not something nebulous like, "I want to get healthy someday." Research backs this up: "future health benefits, such as disease prevention, are too abstract to overcome people's inertia and hectic schedules."[26] If we can define a more long-term goal that meets a constant need, we can merge our lower brain's need for survival, our upper brain's need for planning, and our middle brain's need to feel good.

The result is your Joy Goal. Jesus had His Joy Goal: reconcile us to Him. The Father saw a need, and Jesus made a way through the cross. You might already have a Joy Goal, a lifelong purpose that you are focused on. Great! Keep that in mind, and you can fine-tune it for your season. What is your current season of life? Are you a student with three years left, a mom of littles, stuck in between jobs, heartbroken after a relationship gone sour? Now picture the end of your season, whether it's graduation, kids going to kindergarten, landing a job, or being single and thriving. What is your prize at the end? God wants to give us more than we can ask or imagine, so let's meet Him in the middle and envision the most outrageous, wonderful outcome we can possibly think of, no obstacles in sight. Be as daring and detailed as you can be.

> *Example: My season of life is having two small children in a new house. My Joy Goal is that by the time my oldest daughter goes to kindergarten, I will be present to train her up in love and nourish our youngest, have the basement finished so my husband can play music and I can train others, and publish a book.*

Write yours down here:

_____

_____

_____

_____

_____

_____

_____

_____

_____

_____

How Can You Get to Your Joy Goal?

> *"Most of us have two lives. The life we live,*
> *and the unlived life within us. Between*
> *the two stands Resistance."*[27]
> STEVEN PRESSFIELD

Whether your Joy Goal is to climb a mountain with your best friend, or something completely sedentary like creating an online course, moving your body is an essential component of the joy equation. Once we have moved out what we do not need, and pinpointed what we do, the next step is to map out the way to get there. Just as my husband and I had to clear trees in the way of our trail, we might need to break off old habits on the way to a Joy Goal.

Each habit consists of a loop with three parts: a cue, a routine, and a reward. The reward is what we aim for. It is the missing piece we need to complete the joy loop, and ingrains positive habits through conditioning. This is why defining our Joy Goal is so important—the perceived reward determines our daily decisions. Each time we feel a need, our brain recalls the pathway we took for this same situation. This is why we go to a familiar restaurant when we're hungry, or watch reruns of a favorite show when we need to relax.

The body is very efficient: the more the brain can parcel together similar situations and decisions, the less energy it will expend. One of the ways it does this is through bundling associations (like defining fitness as something to be avoided) and taking well-worn paths made through consistent behaviors. Think about the last time you felt tired, but it was the middle of the workday or the kids were acting wild, and you couldn't take a nap. Which way did you choose?

If this is not a habit you want to continue, how do you shut down old those pathways? Instead of focusing on restriction, make decisions in alignment with your Joy Goal to define that pathway and make it easier to take the next time. The less we take a previous thought way, the weaker it becomes. The saying, "If you don't use it, you lose it," becomes your best friend in habit breaking.

Since our thoughts are the bridge between our emotions and our actions, visualizing the reward is the start of laying a new neurological pathway to get to a Joy Goal.

Envision your Joy Goal. At the end of your season, what would your ideal day look like? Write it down, and be as detailed as possible, answering questions like:

1. When do you wake up?

_____

2. How do you feel physically?

_____

3. Do you have a plan for the day? What is it?

_____

4. How do you feel mentally?

_____

5. Whom would you spend time with?

_____

6. How do those people make you feel emotionally?

_____

7. At the end of the day, what can you give thanks for?

_____

8. How do you feel spiritually?

_____

Joy is the light at the end of the tunnel that shows us the way, and compassion for others (including yourself) is the heat that gets us moving. Whom is this Joy Goal for?

_____

_____

_____

See if you can relate with any of the current needs, and highlight the corresponding Joy Goal that encompasses your ideal day. Each intrinsic motivator is linked to a specific pathway, explained in Chapters Three to Seven, designed to connect you to the Lord, your ultimate source of joy. If you're not sure, take the quiz at the end of this chapter.

Current Need	Joy Goal	I will take the way of the
Feeling unworthy	Confident	Looker: look to Jesus for confidence
Feeling stressed	Peaceful	Freebird: meet with Jesus for peace
Feeling isolated/ underchallenged	Victorious	Warrior: join with Jesus' body for victory
Feeling worn out	Energized	Hero: be filled with Jesus for Kingdom effectiveness
Feeling unhealthy	Healthy	Keeper: listen to Jesus to care for the body

How to Use This Book

Once you have identified which motivator will best lead you to your Joy Goal, by taking the quiz below, read the corresponding chapter. Then read the remaining motivator chapters. There might be another motivator that you can relate to depending on your mood, or one that will help you relate with someone else in your life.

I had one client who was dreading going snow skiing with her husband for vacation. He saw it as a challenge, and wanted to put her on a training plan to help her succeed. He is a Warrior. She, on the other hand, did not so much care for timing or testing her potential. She loved skiing because it made her feel good that she was taking care of her body in such a fun way. She is a Keeper. Neither motivation is "correct," but highlights their unique wiring. The last chunk of the book will help you put your Joy Goal into action.

Here's a quick recap:

Assess (feel)
1.   What is not working out in my fitness journey? Prayerfully move out what you do not need.

Ask (think)
2.   What am I searching for? Write down your Joy Goal according to what you need.
3.   Which way do I take to reach my Joy Goal? Choose and read Chapters Three to Seven.

Act (do)
4.   Chapter Eight: By faith, figure out what you need to do for discipline, and what you want to do by design.
5.   Chapter Nine: Take the next step. Reverse engineer your goal and break it down into smaller steps. Learn how to modify as needed.

6. Chapter Ten: Stay focused on joy. Identify enemies of distraction and shame, grow in patience, and surround yourself with reminders.

Bonus Chapter: Quick ways to spark joy in survival mode

As Dr. Ashley Null observed as the basis of behavior in the Common Book of Prayer, "What the heart loves, the will chooses, and the mind justifies."[28] This is a process of heart reorientation, not behavior modification. We often start out like moths, attracted to the light of joy, constantly reaching out for what's missing. But once we connect with the source of our heart's desires, we become the light of joy, and can reach out to others. Moving the feet will become an overflow of a joyful heart.

Know Your Season

The hike with my husband was my bucket-list item for our vacation together, but it was fall and cool enough for me to enjoy it. It was the right season. As I write this, I am in a season of swimming. I used to hate swimming! Every childhood summer, we had to tread water for two minutes to be permitted in our neighborhood pool's deep end. I cried every time. Just imagine me floundering, only my face above water, while my friends cheered me on so I could play pool games with them during the summer. How embarrassing! And, looking back, how lovely of them. Today, my season is pregnancy. Thankfully, I have since learned new swimming skills (i.e. how to relax and how to breathe) and really enjoy the deep end. When summer is over and the humidity doesn't make my hair stick to my face as soon as I step outside into the Georgia heat, I'll go back to walking everywhere around town. When I need a challenge, I'll show up to boxing class or sign up for a 5K. When I need to relax and unwind, I go to yoga or play my favorite dance music. To everything, there is a season. What is yours?

The Loop Exercise

The next time you go on a hiking loop, walk from your house and back, or travel around a track, think about how you are changed each time you complete a full revolution. The scenery on the outside might seem the same, but on the inside you have strengthened the circular network within your body to bring your systems back to homeostasis faster the next time. Imagine that each loop is a day in the life of walking with Jesus, and each day brings you closer to home, closer to the joy of His full presence forever.

Your Fitness Motivator Quiz

After each of the multiple choice questions, there is a number in parenthesis. Pick the one that *most* fits you right now. Keep a tally of those numbers to get your score.

1. **Which fitness headline appeals to me most?**
   a. "Best Circuit Workout: Think You Can Handle It?" (4)
   b. "Strong and Sexy" (1)
   c. "Energy Blast" (3)
   d. "Instant Calm" (2)
   e. "Nourish Your Body" (5)

2. **At the beginning of the day, I struggle with:**
   a. Choosing which awesome thing I want to do (4)
   b. My mile-long to-do list (3)
   c. My reflection in the mirror (1)
   d. Stress (2)
   e. Thinking about how to prevent injury (5)

3. **I choose a workout based on:**
   a. The epic factor: if I can learn a new skill or explore new territory, I'm in. (4)
   b. A science-backed plan proven to boost immunity and banish disease. (5)
   c. How many calories does it burn? Will it fix my trouble zones? (1)
   d. How peaceful I will feel. (2)
   e. How efficient it will be: What workout has the most multitasking moves in 20 minutes? (3)

4. *My exercise tipping point is:*
- a. Seeing pictures of myself (1)
- b. Needing to let off some steam (2)
- c. Overhearing a friend talk about how awesome their group workout is (4)
- d. Feeling guilty over skipping a planned workout (3)
- e. Getting less-than-ideal lab results back from the doctor (5)

5. *I avoid exercise because:*
- a. It's too painful. (5)
- b. There are too many people at the gym and I'm not fit enough yet. (1)
- c. The last plan was too rigid. (2)
- d. It's boring and not challenging enough by myself. (4)
- e. I'm taking care of everyone else and don't have time. (3)

6. *Deep down, I want to:*
- a. Have energy to focus on what's important. (3)
- b. Shift my focus from my body to other parts of my life. (1)
- c. Be a ninja of tranquility with a balanced, strong interior that isn't shaken by external circumstances. (2)
- d. Be a positive example for the next generation. (5)
- e. Know I am capable, powerful, and connected with others. (4)

7. *I like this feeling after a workout:*
- a. Pumped up, walking tall (1)
- b. Energized, with more to give (3)
- c. Sweaty high fives (4)

d. Settled and put together (2)

e. To hear, "Great job today!" (5)

8. My usual long-term fitness goal is motivated by:

    a. Training for a race, competition, or other challenge (4)

    b. A special event, like a beach trip, reunion, or wedding (1)

    c. What long-term goal? (2)

    d. Avoiding genetic diseases (5)

    e. A workout plan that fits into my already determined schedule (3)

9. What inspires me to move:

    a. Finding a workout that helps me look like the fitness instructor or superhero on screen (1)

    b. New challenges and friendly competition (4)

    c. Escaping, whether that's through meditation, music, or getting outside (2)

    d. Having a results-based plan with no unnecessary downtime (3)

    e. A health professional keeping me accountable (5)

10. This distracts me, and I think a workout can help!

    a. Aches and pains are annoying, but not something I have time to address. (3)

    b. I'm tired of feeling unhealthy, whether that's from extra weight, fatigue, pain, or other illness. (5)

    c. Overstimulation and overwork. (2)

    d. I can't wait to unlock my hidden potential and be the best I was created to be. (4)

    e. Tight-fitting clothes makes me unable to focus on the rest of my life. (1)

SCORING

10-17	Looker
18-25	Freebird
26-34	Hero
35-42	Warrior
43-50	Keeper

ASK:
Which Way Will You Take?

Chapter Three

The Looker: Feel Confident

Our five-year anniversary trip was my husband's tipping point. We ate our way through New York City: savored pizza with crispy crust, devoured toasted bagels piled high with strawberry cream cheese, and drooled over authentic Italian paninis. We may have walked ten miles a day and offset a few calories, but on our return trip, hubby took one look at our pictures and decided he needed to start working out.

He's a big fan of comics and anything Marvel, so when an office mate told him about an online workout program designed to chisel his body into Peter Quill from *Guardians of the Galaxy,* he signed up and got to work.

As I write this, one year after his program start, I can proudly say he dutifully sticks to his workout routine, has lost twenty pounds, and has also drastically changed his eating habits. I say the word "proudly," knowing that I had nothing to do with his success. I tried everything from subliminal messages to blatant requests to join me at the gym, but as the Lord reminded me yet again, I didn't need to change him to be like me, but to support him to be more of himself. I've noticed that relationships function like partnering muscle groups: to curl a weight, the bicep contracts and the tricep relaxes. I needed to relax to let him flex.

If there were any lingering doubts about his intentions, this scenario convinced me. One night after dinner, I offered him a brownie or a sugar-free cocoa energy bite. The old husband would have chosen brownie, no question. The new husband took the energy bite and dismissed the brownies with a wave of his hand declaring, "I can't eat that fluff! I'm trying to build muscles." That caught me by surprise because I definitely chose brownies. He had been transformed! I was impressed... and perplexed.

Overeating is my biggest obstacle to living well, but food was no longer a temptation for him. What was this new motivation that prompted such attractive self-control?

He had one focus: muscles. He pictured the body he wanted to build, and sugar had no part in it. Could it be that his incentive to achieve a certain look was a positive factor for long-term health? Could I learn something eternally joyful from his desire to look a certain way?

Why We Need to Look Good

From an athletic perspective, seeing is the precursor to doing. We have an evolutionary trait that lets us observe others and learn from them without actually moving. This way, we can calculate their potentially fatal errors and avoid repeating them. We see Junior doing a cartwheel off a cliff, and we know he took one step too many. Our brain has now captured that movement warning. What this means for our fitness endeavors is that we can start picking up a new sport by watching a champion, we can prepare our bodies for action by visualizing, and we can reinforce the budding neural pathways laid down by observation with doing.

Seeing not only helps us prevent death, but procreate for more life. Good looks are an evolutionary adaptation. We are attracted to healthy characteristics in others (a noticeable lack of disease, a symmetric frame, reproductive age) so we can be fruitful and multiply with the strongest genes. We subconsciously associate beauty with health. However, cultural beauty does not always coincide with posterity and our priorities get skewed. Societal beauty is perpetuated by what our eyes continually take in, and the standard shifts with each generation. What we see shapes who we are, and in turn, influences how we think we should be shaped, but we may not even realize what we are absorbing: "only eight percent of an image's message is received by the conscious mind. This means that we are vastly unaware of the impact an image has on our consciousness!"[29]

We may see a movie star and tuck the image away in our lower subconscious brain, not realizing that this picture contributes to our own visual archetype of the flawless body, the "right" way to look. This image comes into full view as we stand in the three-way mirror in the Target dressing room, completely unaware of how just subconsciously absorbed the blown-up advertisements of smiling supermodels that greeted us on the way in. The cumulative media messages build up and weigh us down (and make us buy more to change ourselves into their ideal image). And we wonder why our slumped-over reflection looks so joyless.

Find Confidence in Challenges

People who self-objectify are the least likely to stick with exercise. While the Looker is motivated by external appearances, the path to joy goes much deeper and is inherently rooted in the confidence of Christ. If the Looker wants to succeed long-term, they need to start from the outside and work our their way in to complete their joy and sustain their Joy Goal.

Maybe you despise what you see in the mirror because you have been rejected, feel less than, or hopeless, thinking that past failures determine your future. You need to be built up and remember who you are. If confidence defines what you need now, you can achieve this feeling by doing challenging exercises that increase the happy neurochemicals of serotonin and endorphins, which create a positive perspective. The key is to challenge yourself in a safe environment, and experience the joy that comes with confidence in conquering something new. If you want more details, Chapter Eight will guide you into more specific exercises.

Every road to gaining confidence has a few hurdles in the way. To a Looker who lacks confidence, a tall hurdle is intimidating. She might get discouraged by its height and walk away from the race. But not you! You are going to train for these hurdles and leap over them like you're on camera. After getting over these hurdles, keep reading to discover how to complete your joy with endurance for the long run.

Hurdle #1

> **Tight-fitting clothes make you unable to focus on your day, let alone your long-distance Joy Goal.**

Leap for Joy: *You wear the clothes, the clothes don't wear you.* If something fits too tight in the dressing room, remove the judgment and take it off because it's not right for you.

A friend recently lost some weight, and after commenting that her main motivation was a pair of fancy-print leggings, I was intrigued. She shares her story here:

> *I found someone who basically kicked me in the rear about coming to a clothing sale, and around the same time, I found myself in the Bible more. I went to the sale and tried some clothes on and realized that while I may not be skinny, I wasn't happy in my clothes and I just didn't know it yet. Afterwards, I bought a few things and went home and gave away three garbage bags of clothes. Once I started dressing for my body type more and spending time in the Bible more, my confidence grew and it was almost like God was saying, "You are beautiful." I started being more mindful about how my body felt when I ate a certain food. Yes, God made me with a slow metabolism and big bones. Yes, I may never fit into a single digit size of clothing. But, he made me beautiful. -Marie*

Tight clothes feel like an accusation, baggy clothes feel like hiding, but clothing that fits your body feels like permission to be you. Let your clothes reflect God's acceptance of you, and let your joy light shine! And as you speak truth as armor over your heart, put the right work out clothes on your body for the activity at hand. Even when you don't feel like an athlete, putting on the clothes of a gold medalist draws out the Warrior in you, equipped to put up a fight for your Joy Goal.

Hurdle #2

**Comparing yourself to others in the gym
or your ideal weight on the scale.**

Leap for Joy: *Don't compare yourself with creation; claim the Creator's love.* The scale has an infamous reputation for measuring health, but there are two sides to every scale. You probably use a digital scale that lights up with a number as you stand on it, but think of an old-fashioned balance beam scale with weights on one side to measure the contents of the other side. Now think of yourself on one side. Whom are you putting on the other side of the scale? Whom are you comparing yourself to? I asked a few friends if they ever exercise to achieve a certain look, and how that has turned out for them. One woman responded:

> *When have I not worked out to achieve a certain shape or look? That has always been the goal. A goal I have never had even one benefit from. Because, every time, I get discouraged. With that goal, I am never satisfied—it doesn't happen fast enough. I don't look as good as that gal over there. She is always going to be better than me. So I give up... until the next time I feel like "getting into shape." -Caroline*

There is no human scale where we will measure up. If you are caught in a comparison trap, I would recommend banishing

the scale. Replace it with a throne. There is only room for one
to sit on a throne, there is only one King, and it is not another
person (including ourselves). If we focus on trying to improve
our own outer appearances, we must have someone or something
else to compare us to, because we are created beings. Only the
 uncreated one, the Creator of all things, is self-defining and able
to exist without the need to compare His value to another. It is
impossible for Him to become jealous of another because He is
matchless. Instead, He is jealous for us because He loves us. He
knows the only way we will see our value and experience the joy
of confidence is when we see ourselves as His. Caroline continues:

> *God is giving me new eyesight in my views about how I
> look, so that when I work out, I do it because it makes me
> healthy, stronger, more positive. And I believe that pleases
> Him, because then I am more able to live as He desires for
> me—to be used as a light to others. But it all goes back to
> a changing mindset...a refocus on Him, not me. Not on my
> troubles, not on my emotions, not on the other "perfect"
> women at the gym. I am His and He knows me by name.
> This is my new gym mantra.*

That sounds like a great Joy Goal mantra, too!

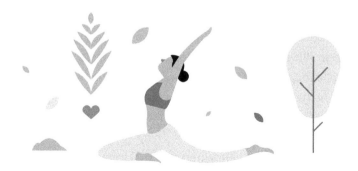

Do you have a truth statement you speak over yourself before, during, or after a workout? You can find the Looker's joy declaration at the end of this chapter.

_____

_____

_____

_____

_____

Hurdle #3

You choose workouts based on how many calories they will burn or which trouble spots they will fix.

Leap for Joy: *Redirect your focus from quantity to quality.* Instead of looking at numbers, visualize your Joy Goal and the confidence you want to achieve. If you want an objective form of measurement, plot a scale from 1-4 for each workout. The lower end is the feeling that you're unworthy and want to hide behind doors or ripped abs. Four is feeling like you're more than a conqueror in Christ. Keep this chart in a spot where you plan your next workout (e.g. a planner, an office bulletin board, next to your gym bag), and record your number before and after.

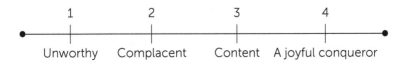

| 1 | 2 | 3 | 4 |
| Unworthy | Complacent | Content | A joyful conqueror |

Make this an experiment: record your measurements for
a workout you don't enjoy, but focuses on calorie burn.
Then, pick an activity that you enjoy doing. Don't keep
track of anything except how you feel before, during, and
after. Which one results in a score of 4, or closest to it?
Keep that exercise in mind for Chapter Nine when you plan
out your Joy Goal.

Hurdle #4

Avoiding public places to exercise because of how you look.

Leap for Joy: *Find a welcoming space.* Some clients pay me to
come and train them at their homes because they don't want
to be seen at the gym, which can feel like intimidating places
for those who don't look the part of a conventionally fit person.
Respondents to a National Institutes of Health survey said being
"too fat" was a barrier for physical activity.[30] I think every gym
should be filled with people of all shapes and sizes, to represent
humanity's truly diverse landscape.

Comedian Jim Gaffigan shares how comfortable he is at his
gym: "Sure my Y doesn't have some of the amenities, but it also
doesn't have the normal health club distractions. I don't have to
deal with loud music or people that are in shape. I walk around
my Y and I'm like, 'You know what? I'm doing okay.'" This sketch
may be part of a stand-up routine, but he's speaking the truth!
He even goes so far as to say, "The most annoying are those
people in exceptionally good shape at the gym. I'm like 'What
are you doing here? You're done.'" "In shape" is not any one
shape, despite how we might peg regular gym goers. You can
begin making your own gym a welcoming space by looking past
appearances and appreciating each person just as they are. Or,

feel free to ditch your current gym for a workout space with the most hospitable, joyful training environment for everyone involved. Your "gym" can simply be a space with another person whom you trust to love and respect you, no matter how you look.

Hurdle #5

If you see someone's body type you like in the gym, on social media, or on screen, you stalk their workouts to discover what they are doing so you can copy them.

Leap for Joy: *Guard your heart by guarding your eyes.* Studies from 2016 show that use of any social networking site was connected to increased disordered eating and body dissatisfaction.[31] When looking through your social media feed, watching a movie, or sharing a weight machine with an attractive person, ask yourself these questions:

- What are you seeing?
- What are they saying?
- What are they selling?
- What are you thinking?

Do your thoughts reflect Colossians 3:12, that you are God's chosen one, holy and beloved? If not, unfollow the person, don't see the movie, or go to a different workout room until the boundary around your heart is firm enough to rebound any identity-destroying thoughts.

Hurdle #6

You double-up your workouts in preparation for a special event, like a beach trip, reunion, or wedding.

Leap for Joy: *Make every day a special event*, because you're alive and loved. Instead of going all in for a short season and then burning out, choose consistency over intensity. Find ways to fold more movement into your everyday life. Try choosing one activity a week as your "bucket-list item." If you're not sure what you like to do, head to Chapter Eight for ideas. Movement can become a vacation you look forward to each week, rather than using exercise to prepare for a one-time event. If there are 52 Saturdays in a year, think of it as having 52 vacations!

More Than Skin Deep

You may be able to leap for joy over small hurdles, but your path may have painfully deep chasms that threaten to pull you under. My friend Olivia courageously shared her story of exercise and body image:

> *I was sexually abused from ages seven to eleven by four different people. As a result of others giving me physical attention, I formed my identity around body image. I wanted to make sure I always looked good, worked out twice a day, and thought I was doing it because I was healthy. I loved working out, but if I didn't, I felt like a bum, like my body was getting fat. There was no grace whatsoever. It made me feel shameful.*
>
> *My turning point was when I went through a sexual abuse class. A lot of the sexually abused women were over-weight or had eating disorders. God showed me that even though I didn't have an eating disorder, I had a distorted image because of my past. He opened my eyes, planted a seed of awareness, and started changing me.*
>
> *Previously, if woke up at 4 a.m., I would work out. Now if I wake up that early, I spend time with God and don't work out (unless God wants me to). I began working out less and trusting Him more, going from two-a-day workouts to exercising three to four times a week. I gave the time that I worked out with God to sit in His presence. I*

*listened to Him say that I'm beautiful and that I didn't need
to get my identity from my past abuse, but from His love.*

Whether you can relate with Olivia's story or not, each of our
roots of shame go way back to the Garden of Eden. The book
of Genesis shares our origin story: Adam and Eve were created
naked, but they were unashamed. It is only when they sinned
that they became self-aware. They *felt* naked because sin separated them from God and stripped the comforting covering of
God's presence. The root of a self-conscious body is an exposed
heart, but a secure heart is a confident body. When God sent
them out of the Garden of Eden to protect them from living in
sin forever, God covered them in animal skins. It was a sign that
God Himself would sacrifice His own body to cover our shame.

Complete Your Joy by Being Covered in Christ

If the Looker is consumed with shame and focus on self, he
misses out on the big picture. A moment of confidence after
lifting weights is a shadow of the never-fading confidence in
Christ. Looking up from himself to the Lord will help him not
only feel the joy he craves now, and help him reach his Joy Goal
later, but free him to look to others and give them the confidence
of being loved for who they are.

The Father knows how much we depend on sight, and gave
us the gift of the incarnation, God in the flesh, a God whom we
could see and touch and follow. Since He has risen to the right
hand of the Father, we can no longer see Him by looking with
our eyes, but through the eyes of faith. And in many ways, not
being bound by sight is even better. We learn to lean not on our
own vision, but in His omnipresent Spirit. Does it even matter
what Jesus looked like, and did his appearance affect how He
saw others? *another verse in gospel says Jesus wasn't particularly*

Interestingly, one of the only verses that mentions the phys- *physically*
ical appearance of Jesus compares Him to a precious plant in *attractive in a great way*

a harsh land. I'm picturing dry, fractured ground with no veg-
etation to cover it, when suddenly, a surprising sapling of joy
sprouts through a tiny crack: "My servant grew up in the LORD's
presence like a tender green shoot, like a root in dry ground.
There was nothing beautiful or majestic about his appearance,
nothing to attract us to him" (Isaiah 53:2 NLT). Jesus's entrance
was not a big premiere. There were no spotlights or camera
flashes, only advance reviews that He wouldn't be winning any
awards for best picture.

Do you think there was any kind of conversation around what
kind of body Jesus would have when He came to Earth? Jesus
could have selected His physical attributes and made Himself
with a "natural" athletic build, posing just so, with His carpentry
hammer like Thor. He could have made life easy on Himself,
because popular belief is that life is easier for beautiful people.
None of the gorgeous celebrities who grace the red carpets of the
Grammys have any problems, and all yours will go away once
you can fit into your skinny jeans, or once you can get rid of that
flabby midsection. Or at least those are the lies the enemy wants
us to believe. In Ezekiel 28:17, God explains Satan's history:
"Your heart was proud because of your beauty; you corrupted
your wisdom for the sake of your splendor. I cast you to the
ground; I exposed you before kings, to feast their eyes on you."
And isn't that exactly what the enemy tried to do to Jesus? To
throw Him down, uncover Him, consume Him?

Except this is Jesus's story, and Jesus is the one who writes
the ending: He was not thrown down. He came down. He con-
cealed His beauty and humbled himself to the point of the cross,
using foolish things to shame the wise and weak things to shame
the powerful. He was rejected by His own people, yet He was
the desire of all nations. He attracted sinners, not because of his
outward beauty, but because of His unparalleled compassion
and authority. No one took his life, but he gave his life over,
and allowed himself to be stripped naked and mocked by the
crowds. He was raised up, on a cross, and laid down in a grave.

They tried to bury him, not knowing he was a seed. And three days later, like a bright plant out of the dark dirt, He burst forth into eternal life!

If you feel unworthy and want to stay in the shadows, that is not from the Lord. Satan fell and wants to take you down with him. You may want to look good so others will like you because they like what they see. But Jesus sees you. And He likes what He sees. And as you slowly lift your head to meet His gaze, you reflect His glory. And that, my friends, is true radiance.

You Are Chosen, Holy, and Beloved

Movement uncovers your confidence in Christ.

We call this motivator "The Looker" for several reasons:

1. Its definition in the early 1900s was: "a very attractive person."
2. It means a person who looks.

You can only believe #1 if you have your focus right for #2.

This truth is based on Colossians 3:12, so let's dig in, and visualize where you want to resurface on the other side of your Joy Goal.

> *"Put on then, as God's chosen ones, holy and beloved, compassionate hearts, kindness, humility, meekness, and patience." Colossians 3:12*

Truth #1: You are already chosen. No need to shrink or build your body for anyone else to pick you as a spouse, a friend, a trainer, a teammate. The King of the world chooses you, royal daughters and sons. Come join the family.

Truth #2: You are holy and beloved. *Holy* means set apart. If you don't fit the mold of the miniscule percentage of "fit body"

Google images, good. You aren't supposed to. You are fit for Him, but you are not to fit in. You are to be set apart for the body of Christ because you are beloved. *Beloved* in the Greek is always defined by God. Being holy and beloved is conforming to the image of Christ, who is the the Holy one of God (Mark 1:24) and the Father's beloved (Matthew 3:17). God already made you in His image, so you can rest in that.

Truth #3: You have a right, an obligation to consistency as it appeals to your need for things to look as they are, to put on the part of one chosen, holy, and beloved.

We cannot add anything to the Scriptures, but we can "adorn the teachings of God our Saviour"[32] by doing them. Adorn your heart with action. Test your thoughts and be aware of your inner dialogue. Would you say to someone else what you are saying to yourself? Are your hidden thoughts ones of compassion, kindness, humility, meekness, and patience? Practice these virtues for yourself as an expression of how God loves you. They say that seeing is believing, but acting your belief is more powerful.

Practice compassion:
We are called as Christians to practice compassion to those who are destitute, afflicted, and hard-pressed. When I hear clients say they want to lose weight, sometimes it's simply for health reasons, and other times, they can mean they want to be respected, loved, seen, and free from fear of others and hate of oneself. This sounds like someone who needs a hug, not a killer workout. Whenever you're tempted to insult a part of your body that has been squeezed, scarred, or stretched, lay a hand of blessing on it instead, in Jesus' name.

Practice kindness:
Kindness is doing what is eternally good and fit for you. This can go either way: if your systems are feeling sluggish, the kind thing

may be to go and move. If your spirit is feeling downtrodden, you might need to swap out the boxing session for restorative yoga to recover your joy.

Practice humility:

> *The old humility was a spur that prevented a man from stopping; not a nail in his boot that prevented him from going on. For the old humility made a man doubtful of his efforts, which might make him work harder. But the new humility makes a man doubtful about his aims, which will make him stop working altogether.*
> GK CHESTERTON [33]

Put aside the false humility that you are better off hiding in your house, and put on the humility that follows Jesus anywhere, even going to a new class at the gym, by yourself, because He always goes first. He is your confident leader!

Practice meekness:
The meek shall inherit the earth. The meek do not seize control of what they want through visual seduction, but by gentleness of character. Meekness is not shrinking back, but putting your trust forward in the Lord that He will glorify you at the right time.

Practice patience:
Patience is being transformed from one degree of glory to another, one day at a time. We are transformed from seeing with our eyes to seeing with our hearts. We become who we are not by each pound lost, but by each step of faith taken. If you feel like you've tried and failed and feel worthless, try again with Jesus. Renew your hope not in the program results, but in the resurrection power.

Joy Gifts of The Looker

Our image-oriented minds and resulting emotions are part of your natural design: "50% of the brain is dedicated to vision. How you look plays a large role in how you feel."[34] Satisfaction with aesthetics is also necessary for the development of our inner being: "And when people cease to be surrounded by beauty, they cease to hope. They internalize the message of their eyes and ears, the message that whispers that they are not worth very much, that they are in effect less than fully human."[35] Surrounding yourself with beauty draws out your inner joy!

Even if you don't change your appearance one bit, exercise will make you appreciate what you already have. A study reported that exercise does not improve body image, but increasing frequency and intensity improves self-esteem, perceived self-efficacy, and increases the chance of establishing a lifelong healthy habit of exercise.[36] You might be surprised how much better you feel about yourself with a regular fitness routine in view of the Lord. Moving for joy will not only help you love yourself as God does, but help you love others. Think back to who your Joy Goal is for, then read the list below with them in mind:

- **You bring out beauty:** The Looker sees hidden potential and puts it on display. She does not shrivel in shame over her body, but takes joy in how God made her. The Looker dresses herself in strength and dignity, always looking for ways to brighten the world and bring heaven's beauty to Earth.

  Share this joy gift by calling out the goodness in others. Do you notice beauty in someone else? Give thanks to God for that gift to your eyes; simply pray "glory" to cover them in confidence (especially if you are running fast past them), and consider telling them what they may not see. You can be their God mirror—the person to show them what He sees! In turn, what does God like about you? Praise Him for making you fearfully and wonderfully.

- **You are willing to invest:** The Looker wants the outside to reflect the inside: holy and beloved. He knows each person is set apart for special use, that gold is refined in the fire, and he's willing to endure the pain of discipline and invest his resources for purity— "no extra spiritual fat, no parasitic sins."[37]

    Enhance this joy gift by being faithful in the small things, and see what God does in and through you as you walk toward your Joy Goal.

Weight loss by itself can feel selfish, but losing shame and being covered in confidence affects everyone around you. This message helps my own heart when I'm feeling inferior, but it also strengthens my marriage. As for my husband, I want to look at him now more than ever. It's not just the way I can wrap my arms around his tight waist or how he lifts me up with his strong arms. It's the way he lifts his head higher and walks taller with confidence. As his wife, I feel like I can trust him more, and that makes me more confident in trusting his words, when he says to me, "I love you. You are beautiful." It's almost as if those words were coming from the Lord himself, and I raise my own head in response.

Exercise:

Let's walk in the confidence of the King and turn "looking good" into a verb. First, slide your chin backwards so that your ears line up over your shoulders. Don't let your crown drop. Next, practice looking long-term for God's eternal purposes by looking at things far away. Our eyes have muscles too, and need to be stretched. The best way to do that is to do the 20-20-20 exercise. Take a break from looking at close-range objects every twenty minutes, and look at something at least twenty feet away for twenty seconds. This will reduce your risk of myopia, or nearsightedness, and improve your vision.

The Looker Quick Reference Guide

When you need to remember what gets you going, refer to the statements below:

Looker motivation: Enjoying the Lord through exercise builds unchangeable confidence.

Joy Declaration: "I am holy, beloved, and chosen in Christ. I will lift my crown, move for joy, and walk worthy of the Lord."

Looker prayers to be used for exercise:
- "You love me beyond looks."
- "Eyes on You."
- "Show me Your glory."

If you identify as a Looker, you may skip to Chapter Eight to begin building your Joy Goal for confidence!

Chapter Four

The Freebird: Relieve Stress

It was Christmas Eve, and I had a perfect plan for the whole family: we would eat breakfast, let our two-year-old open one gift, and then I could have a rejuvenating exercise session by myself. Our daughter played with her new kinetic sand for more than ten minutes, which is an eternity in toddler time. The morning was off to a good start! I began gearing up for my run, expecting my husband to take over. He was on his computer and thought she would be fine playing on her own.

I started feeling resentful. *I* spent time playing with her, and now it was *his* turn. I was clearly jealous of his ability to have free time. She would be fine on her own, but I thought she needed a constant playmate. Since he wasn't playing with her, then by process of elimination, it had to be me. My narrow-minded logic arrived at one conclusion: I couldn't go on a run. I felt trapped, and I must have started to hyperventilate. I voiced my mental record of rights—how I play with her *all the time* (marriage tip: *never* use absolutes), and that good dads played with their kids on Christmas Eve. He just looked at me and told me to go on my run.

"But, you…" I protested.

"Go on," He motioned me out the door.

I went off in a huff. He knew I would feel better after I could work it out with the Lord. Looking back, I see now that I may have overreacted just a bit.

This is like when kids start whining for no apparent reason, and you tell them to go play outside and they come back ten minutes later, heaving, covered in dirt, but happy as can be, offering things like, "Would you like a foot rub after tea time, Mum?" (in this purely fictional representation, the polite kid has a delightful British accent). When I threw my little adult tantrum, my downstairs brain took over, and I couldn't think clearly or compassionately. I was not joyful because I was not at peace. My mind felt like a ransacked room with no quiet place to sit down.

I remembered reading about a movement anger-management solution in *Whole Brain Child*, and found that it works for adults, too:

> *"Research has shown that bodily movement directly affects the brain chemistry. So when one of your children has lost touch with his upstairs brain, a powerful way to him regain balance is to have him move his body...However you do it, the point is to help your child regain some sort of balance and control by moving their body, which can remove blockages and pave the way for integration to return."*[38]

Finding this sense of balance is exactly what the Freebird craves! Anger, stress, and overwhelm send us on an endless negative feedback loop, which in turn leads to physical dysfunction[39]:

But movement helps circulate oxygen, reintegrate our brains, and relax the resting tension of our muscles, which breaks the stress hold over our bodies. Statistically speaking, exercise reduces symptoms of anxiety by more than 50 percent.[40]

What kind of exercise helps restore the flow of joy? Engaging in any kind of mindful activity induces peace by releasing GABA neurochemicals to induce a sense of calm, endocannabinoids for a feeling of bliss, and endorphins to relieve stress. It can be yoga, but it doesn't have to be. In fact, if anxiety levels are sky high, then high intensity exercise makes a good match to out-compete the anxious physical symptoms.

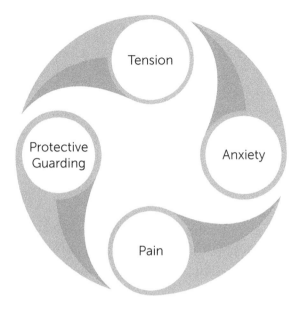

In any case, the activity needs to be something that can be mentally pull together an individual throughout the movement. We will run through more specifics throughout the chapter.

How the Freebird Endures

Let's hear how Kimberly finds her stress relief in fitness: "I have three boys, and we were home all summer. When I needed time for myself to get my head straight, I would take my kids to the YMCA and settle them into childwatch."

The next part is what completes her joy:

"Then, I would put on my Bethel worship music and go for a thirty-minute walk to clear my head, listen, pray, and finish up with free weights. I've been in a season of wanting that contemplative time. My workouts seem to involve a lot of walking and praying, and if I can fit in free weights or a yoga class, I'll do that too. We're in a really busy season of life, and so for me exercise with the Lord is meeting the need of releasing stress and anxiety. "

The Freebird doesn't need to escape to Tahiti. She can find the refreshment of peace by meeting with the Lord in the temple of her own body. Exercise is one of the best, and cheapest, ways to facilitate that peace. Your quiet time doesn't have to be still time, but it does help to create an environment that allows for a still heart: think slow, mindful movement to get recentered, or going all in to burn off the stress.

Getting Away to Be with the Father

The Bible doesn't mention Jesus getting "stressed," but He was in many stressful situations. Whole towns and villages followed Him for healing, religious leaders publicly opposed Him, and His own friends tried to pressure Him into military rule. Anytime He tried to get some peace and quiet, there was somebody who needed His help or wanted His head. Jesus was God, but He was also man, and He experienced the same survival response mechanisms built in to preserve us when something threatens our well-being. When Jesus needed to unwind, He would walk away from the masses of people to "desolate places," or as the New International Version says, "lonely places" to pray: "But now even more the report about him went abroad, and great crowds gathered to hear him and to be healed of their infirmities. But he would withdraw to desolate places and pray" (Luke 5:15-16).

Jesus wasn't driven away by fear or annoyance. He was motivated by precious communion with His dad. He wasn't merely getting away from the crowds. He was going to be with our Father. The result was always a renewed resolve. His prayer time equipped Him to both rise above the needy mob, and to move toward them as a Shepherd leading stressed-out sheep into a spacious safe haven.

When is the last time you met with the Lord, just you and him? Describe the before and after experience.

_____

_____

_____

_____

_____

How were your stress levels before and after on a scale of overwhelmed to overflowing?

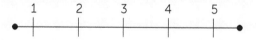

Your Body is a Temple

The Freebird mission:
Get away with God through exercise.

Jesus's prayer hikes not only serve as an example of stress relief, but of the true inner peace, or shalom, that can only be experienced within God's presence. Where can we find God? In the mountains? At a retreat center? Up in the clouds? We can find Him in His temple. His temple is not a building with four walls, but fleshly bodies of faith. Our very body is the meeting space between heaven and Earth. When God says He wants to live with us, He really means it!

Stress makes us feel like we need to get out, but God reminds us He is right here within. Stress makes us chase our tails, but

God's presence reminds us we have had our tail all along. We have had Him all along. It's okay to be in our bodies, because there we can meet with God. The more present we are with Him in the space of our bodies, the safer we feel to be our true selves, and to ditch dogmas that pressure us ino exercising the "right way." Dr. Dwayne Golbek, chiropractor and certified strength and conditioning specialist, explains how grace broke him free to experience the boundless joy of Christ in every available movement:

> I started to get bored with exercise because I had put it into a box, which sucked the joy from it for me and isolated me from others. For example, I didn't understand why I could squat below parallel with no issues, but other people shouldn't because it was 'bad for their knees.' I was listening to all the books, which told me that deadlift was the answer to everything. This rigid attitude restricted my own perspective and put me in conflict with many of my clients.
>
> Around the same time, my wife started to show me some pastors that taught the grace message in its entire truth, which opened up my mind to seeing how the Good News could be translated into everything. My newfound excitement led me to to try different exercises that didn't necessarily have to be in a gym (rock climbing, body weight movements, primitive movements, even just a walk through the woods). I started appreciating EVERY movement for what it was and enjoy a much more functional style of training, that is just as fun as it is challenging.
>
> Now my preferred training style is intuitive movement: doing what makes your body feel good and not forgetting the purpose of fitness, which is to live a happy healthy life, able to continue doing the things you enjoy. I feel closer to God, not only when I squat heavy or finish a seemingly impossible rock climbing route, but also when I take a leisurely walk with my wife and son. I experience joy with the

Lord through fitness in a way that is literally filled with endless opportunities to discover what the body that He created for me can do.

Dwayne brings up an important concept: intuitive training. This style of fitness is not only helpful for the Freebird, but can be used to modify your Joy Goal as needed. You will learn more about how to put this into practice in Chapter Nine.

But what about when we feel too emotionally overwhelmed that we are unable to be still and tune in? The stress of anxiety can feel like frayed live wires, while depression is like a cord cut off from its energy source. Both need a place to connect to restore the flow of joy. Grounding is a great place to start. Grounding, or earthing, is the act of connecting with the electrons on the Earth's surface. It may sound bizarre, but studies have shown that walking barefoot for thirty minutes a day, or connecting to grounded connective systems indoors, shows rapid shifts to a parasympathetic dominance in the nervous system (making you feel more calm), improves heart rate variability (the heart can adapt to stress more quickly), and normalizes muscle tension (releasing overall stress).[41] Another method of grounding that does not include going shoeless involves exercises in mindfulness. When we ground ourselves in the moment, we can find deeper communion with the God of the present.

Instead of rushing through an intense workout to get it over with, try a slower session, like yoga or Pilates, that encourages you to pay attention to your breath and be present in your body. Feel the stretch in your muscles and, yes, the burning sensation when it gets hard. Our primal reaction is to avoid any type of discomfort. Don't try to move past it, or be afraid of it, but make it your focus to simply feel it. I once heard a yoga instructor say, "the most spiritual thing we can say is, 'It feels like this.'"

Feeling somatic signals help you feel emotions, too. You can even practice this by easing into a cool pool without wincing, or turning the shower water colder for a a few seconds. You can start slowly in short intervals to get used to being uncomfortable. Become friends with the sensation as you lean into the solution. As Abraham Lincoln said, "Am I not destroying my enemies when I make friends of them?" By noticing each feeling without judgement, you train yourself to quit assigning moral values to what kind of person you are based on how jiggly your arms feel or how weak your muscles seem during a movement. Conclude each attempt into your own discomfort zone by reaching out to connect your body's physical sensations with the space you find yourself in. Complete the joy circuit by saying thank you to God for giving you that way to interact with His creation.

When you want to practice mindfulness in a workout, use your hand to remind you of the five senses to tune in to. Designate one finger to each sense to attach yourself to the present space. For example:

1. Thumb is feeling: feel the contraction in your calves as you lift up on our toes.
2. Pointer is seeing: Look at your body and at the room around you. Think about how you are the only one who sees yourself from this perspective. What do you see?
3. Middle finger is hearing: Pick out all the sounds around you. What do you hear that you didn't before? Why do you think you tuned it out?
4. Ring finger is smelling: Do you smell sweat? Body odor? Nothing at all? How does this fold into your experience of human movement?
5. Pinky is tasting: You may not be tasting anything, so notice that too. Are you okay with not having food in your mouth? What does it feel like to not notice taste?

The Freebird's Verse

Freebird, let's break down your core verse into manageable steps and let it train you for peace in your next stressful situation.

"Or do you not know that your body is a temple of the Holy Spirit within you, whom you have from God?"
1 Corinthians 6:19

Step 1. Recognize the Stress (Awareness)

"Do you not know…?"

Paul writes to the Corinthian church to remind them that their flesh and blood is a temple of God. It truly is a radical concept to grasp, and we can never hear it enough. We get used to living in our ways. We even get habituated to good things and the joy fades. As the nose gets used to a pleasant aroma and then over time stops sending the brain the good-smell signal, we forget it's even there. We need different stimuli to remind us of the truth of our physical status as temples, whether that is on a different day or in a new way.

It is interesting to note that one of the most effective methods of healing trauma is bodywork. Like laying hands on others for prayer, kind physical touch is healing. It helps to release the stored tension and restores body awareness, as outline in *The Body Keeps the Score*:

> *Mindful touch and movement grounds people and allows them to discover tensions that they may have held for so long that they are no longer even aware of them. When you are touched, you wake up to the part of your body that is being touched. The body is physically restricted when emotions are bound up inside. People's shoulders tighten;*

*their facial muscles tense. They spend enormous energy on
holding back their tears—or any sound or movement that
might betray their inner state.*[42]

If you want more information on this topic, both books, *The
Body Keeps the Score* and *Muscular Retraining for Pain-Free
Living,* contain a wealth of education for how the body stores
stress and different methods of releasing it.[43] The Assess and
Feel part of *Move for Joy* is so essential. We cannot change what
we are not aware of. It is especially helpful for the stressed person
to be reminded of her boundaries to corral the stress. Drawing
the hands across the body is one tactile method of communicat-
ing to ourselves that the lines have fallen in pleasant places.[44]

Increasing awareness exercise:

Sometimes we don't know how to release our bodies without tensing them first and feeling that opposite stimulus.
This exercise is best done lying on the ground. Start with
your feet and clench them as tight as you can for a long
inhale, while keeping the rest of your body relaxed, then
release fully for an extended exhale in an act of surren-
der. When you breathe out, pretend you are fogging up
a mirror, and feel the air expressed from the back of your
throat. Do this for each muscle group, moving to the top of
your body. Which parts feel more relaxed? These might be
areas where you store stress and need more attention.

Step 2: Remove yourself from stress (flight)

"Your body is a temple."

Your body is not an immovable tree or a spineless jellyfish. You have legs to move yourself away from detrimental situations, and integrity to orient you heavenwards. The temple is no longer a stationary structure, but a living, breathing, moving body—*your* body included! If we find ourselves in an oppressive situation, God can deliver us out of it, but we've got to move (Please keep in mind this does not apply to abusive situations. If you're in an abusive situation, please reach out, and get the help you need[45]).

Exodus 14:14 is often quoted in a translation that says, "The LORD will fight for you; you need only to be still," but in other places that word "still" is substituted for "silent," or "hold your peace." It doesn't mean to let the Egyptians, or whatever form of anxiety is on the attack, to capture us, but to have a still, peaceful heart that trusts in the Lord and is ready to follow His command on a dime. This level of trust trains agility—the ability to change directions quickly when needed. In the very next verse, God tells the Israelites to *get going*: "The LORD said to Moses, 'Why do you cry to me? Tell the people of Israel to go forward'" (Exodus 14:15).

When I have found myself in moments of stress, I tend to overthink and overeat instead of obeying the Lord's nudging right away to get going—outside, on a spin bike, whatever I can do in the moment. Moving my body helps me get ahead of my enemies of stress. Sometimes, it can be that simple to let the Lord lead and find peace on the other side.

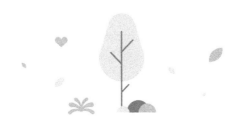

What does He need to deliver you out of?

_____

_____

_____

What Red Sea obstacles are in front of you?

_____

_____

_____

Can you trust God to lead you into the Promised land?
What promises has He given you, and what's the next step
you can take toward them?

_____

_____

_____

_____

Step 3: Release stress from you (fight)

...of the Holy Spirit within you, whom you have from God.

Once you have recognized the source of stress and removed yourself from a harmful situation (even if that's just shutting your eyes to the chaos around you), you can release the stress. Stress, like the money changers that Jesus chased from the temple, is not welcome in the Lord's living temples. Removing the clutter helps usher in your Joy Goal of peace. Exercise has been proven to be one of the best preventative and effective treatments for stress-related mood, sleep, and anxiety disorders, by itself or alongside medication.

- This helped my brother greatly.

When we are stressed, we breathe faster, our hearts beats quickly, and we start sweating. The physiological symptoms of stress are the same, no matter what kind of stress we undergo. Usually, stress arrives from external circumstances that are outside of our control, so when we exercise in the controlled environment of a planned workout fit for our body, we are now the ones in charge of increasing the levels at a beneficial pace. Exercise puts us in power over stress.

When I asked friends on Facebook how they de-stress, the majority of respondents go for a walk. Walking might be the most ancient of exercises. Hippocrates (c. 460 – c. 370 BC), a Greek physician, believed walking is the best medicine. Soren Kierkegaard, a prolific 19th century Danish philosopher and theologian, wrote about the benefits of walking to his favorite niece, Henriette Lund: "Above all, do not lose your desire to walk. Every day, I walk myself into a state of well-being and walk away from every illness. I have walked myself into my best thoughts, and I know of no thought so burdensome that one cannot walk away from it." Walking is the body's most primal movement and naturally realigns us. It doesn't require much planning or forethought, and gets us out of our own heads. Walking, specifically outdoors, offers powerful benefits:

- *Battles disease, depression, and increases positivity:* Sunlight stimulates Vitamin D synthesis, and a small amount of UV exposure reduces risk factors for diseases like multiple sclerosis. Walking outdoors also improves working memory, dampens anxiety,[46] and decreases activity in the part of the brain that centers on repetitive negative emotions.[47]
- *Quicker recovery:* The natural soundscape of the outdoors has been proven to promote faster recovery from physiological stress.[48]
- *Adjust more efficiently:* It's not just the uplifting environmental harmonies that reduces the strain on our body, but also the trees. Trees secrete a substance called phytoncides, which protects the trees from bug enemies while lowering cortisol levels, reducing blood pressure, and slowing heart rates in people.[49]

Wherever you go, be encouraged that God will meet you there: "Where shall I go from your Spirit? Or where shall I flee from your presence? If I ascend to heaven, you are there! If I make my bed in Sheol, you are there!" (Psalm 139:7-8) There is no place that God isn't. Exercise isn't simply a way of escaping from stress, but a way to fly into His arms. You can find peace in His temple.

What types of movement help you release stress?

_____

_____

_____

_____

How can restoring peace help you regain clarity for your
Joy Goal?

_____

_____

_____

_____

_____

Joy Goal Hurdles

In an effort to break free from the stress and find peace, the
Freebird may turn to exercise purely to zone out, get out, or
depend on it to feel better and forget about God's presence. These
hurdles can become sources of stress in themselves and trip up
the Freebird on her way toward true peace. May she open her
wings and fly over each one for joy:

Hurdle #1:

> **_Resistant to new activities. When you need a_**
> **_cognitive break, you tend to run to the same activity_**
> **_to get some refreshment. As a result of wanting to_**
> **_zone out, you stay in your physical comfort zone and_**
> **_miss out on the joy of variety._**

Fly for Joy: A low-barrier activity like walking or running may
be the Freebird's no-brainer solution to stress. But if this is
your only form of exercise, you may be neglecting other areas
of your body, throwing off the peaceful balance. Make it a point
to take care of every part, even when you don't want to. Men
tend to skip lower body exercises while women would rather

skimp on upper body exercise. These are usually weak points for each gender, which is exactly why we need to spend extra care to strengthen them. Men, if you hate squats and lunges, put them at the beginning of your routine or on Mondays when willpower is at its peak. Ladies, do your push-ups. I am a huge fan of push-ups, pull-ups, and progressing them over time. Proverbs 31 does say, "She makes her arms strong!" Make sure to write down your new routine so you won't have to think about it, and can still use fitness as a mental retreat.

Hurdle #2:

> **Inconsistency. If you hardly ever do the same thing
> twice and are always up to try new activities, this
> may give you a well-rounded sense of movement,
> but you may be lacking in the discipline needed
> to keep you on track for your Joy Goal.**

Fly for Joy: On the opposite end of the spectrum, some Freebirds are always looking for fun ways to avoid mediocrity. You want to be *free*, not pinned down by any one program. The hurdle here is that some movements are not right for your body, season, or stage of life. Maybe jumping rope isn't the best exercise postpartum. Perhaps committing to 5:30 a.m. spin class doesn't make sense if you have been assigned the night shift. If you can't remember the last time you kept a workout schedule, it could be time to keep track. Being free is not just about doing what you want, but doing what you need, so you are equipped to do what is best.

Hurdle #3:

> **Expecting endorphins to make everything
> okay. When you go into a workout to restore
> the peace and it doesn't deliver, you might
> be left feeling even worse than before.**

Fly for Joy: *Create space.* Instead of wondering, "How can I feel better?" Ask yourself, "What is the real problem here?" If a lack of exercise is not the problem, it will not serve as a solution. A workout might not make everything better, but going outside for a jog can help create the space needed to gain a broader perspective and get any stuck emotions moving again.

Gifts of the Freebird

You have the gift, not only to be at peace, but to be a peacemaker and bring joy to others.

> ↳ *Exercise may not be the solution to your problem (often it's not), but it gives you space and God, time, to work on your heart.*

- **You have a deep awareness of intimacy with God and know how to access it:** The Freebird knows she does not need to rely on others or uncontrollable circumstances to be at peace. She uses her own body to move away from the fray and get into a place alone with her Heavenly Father.

  Cultivate this gift by planning regular times of movement into solitude, trusting that God will always meet you with His joyful presence, even when you don't feel Him there.

- **You worship with a whole, unhindered heart:** You don't hold anything back. When the Word says to love the Lord your God with all your heart, mind, soul, and strength, you do it with everything you are. You are free to express your need and appreciation for God in a pure posture that overflows straight from your heart through your fingertips:

The Bible describes worship in physical terms. The root meaning for the Hebrew word we translate worship is 'to prostrate.' The word bless literally means 'to kneel.' Thanksgiving refers to 'an extension of the hand.' Throughout Scripture we find a variety of physical postures in connection with worship: lying prostrate, standing, kneeling, lifting the hands, clapping the hands, lifting the head, bowing the head, dancing, and wearing sackcloth and ashes. The point is that we are to offer God our bodies as well as all the rest of our being. Worship is appropriately physical. We are to present our bodies to God in a posture consistent with the inner spirit in worship.[50]

Barring respect for the occasion and place you are in, you feel free to worship God in whatever way He moves you, whether that means sitting, kneeling, stretching, standing, dancing, or running.

Spread the joy: Your purity of worship is contagious to everyone around you. Others will be emboldened to follow God as freely as you, and joy will follow.

While I was out on my Christmas Eve run, I was able to fly from the stress and release it—down to the pavement and up to the skies in prayer. By walking out the door, I separated myself from the situation and stepped out into a bigger world, making my entitled opinions seem small. Running allowed me to wrestle with the Lord within instead of with my husband. Praying actually transforms the brain and promotes love toward others by strengthening "a unique neural circuit that specifically enhances social awareness and empathy while subduing destructive feelings and emotions."[51] This is how I was transformed on the way:

- **Identity:** I am not my husband's Holy Spirit—God is. I am not the lord over my own life—God is. *Who is God telling you He is in the middle of your stress? Who are you in relation to Him?*
- **Compassion:** Once I put myself aside and let the Lord enter in, I was able to step into my husband's shoes and see from his perspective. *When you're having a difficult time loving someone else, how can you put yourself in his or her shoes or see the situation through their eyes?*
- **Priorities:** When I replayed the scenario through my

husband's view, I saw that all he wanted was to do was spend quality time with me. He was keeping himself occupied until I was done with my personal agenda. *How is God shifting your thoughts to align with His design?*

When our thoughts turn into destructive tornadoes, God invites us to come away with Him into the wilderness, just as we are. There He can remind us of our identity in Him, how to love the people He has placed around us, and how to order our lives. By the time I walked back through the door, I felt free from my own need for control. I was at peace, ready to make peace, and we could all enjoy each other's presence because I had reconnected with the Presence within.

Exercise

The sympathetic nervous system, the one that activates adrenaline and a rapid heart beat during times of stress, can be activated by inhaling or taking a few quick inhales to prepare for a competition. Let's take advantage of the partnering system and activate the parasympathetic nervous system (to remember the meaning of this word, I picture a parachute floating down to ground) by focusing on your exhale. Every time you are confronted with a stressful thought, on every long exhale, lift up your hands as as a sign of release and an act of giving every anxiety over to the Lord. Let it be a physical sign of acting out the stress and pushing it away from you.

Freebird Quick Reference Guide

When you need to remember what gets you going, refer to the statements below:

Freebird motivation: Enjoying the Lord through exercise is freedom.

Joy declaration: "I am a temple of the Holy Spirit. I will move for joy to meet God right where I am and find peace."

Freebird prayers to be used for exercise:
- "The Lord is with me, I am with the Lord."
- "Jesus is here."
- "Here I am, Lord."

If you are a Freebird and are ready to put your Joy Goal plan for peace together, skip to Chapter Eight to begin!

Chapter Five

The Hero: Energize

It's 2 p.m., and I just hit my productivity low of the day. So as usual, I stock up on carbs. My real problem is fatigue, but I can't allow myself to take a nap with all the things I need to get done during my daughter's highly unpredictable nap time. For the second week in a row, I go through the motions of portioning out plantain chips and a few pieces of dark chocolate (even though I just finished lunch an hour ago) and settle down for a foggy-headed email session. I feel a quick burst of energy, but it's fleeting, and I feel even more tired. My work is sloppy at best.

Chips and chocolate can only get me so far! I tried to fill the hole of tiredness with carbs instead of the longer-lasting strength of exercise. I should have listened to my recent read *Power of When*. The author advised someone with my chronotype (a chronotype is similar to an early bird or night owl) to exercise in the afternoon to stave off pre-dinner hunger and get that burst of energy that's needed. But chips are way easier (and not to mention tastier) than exercise, and I couldn't answer emails while working out… or could I? What I really wanted was to be efficient with my time so I could serve my family well. I had to find a way to get out of my snack rut.

Why We Need to Be the Hero

In an attempt to save time, I took a shortcut by pushing through my tiredness and stuffing myself full of food so my fatigue signals would stop bothering me. But have you noticed that all the other "time savers" in society actually ramp up the expectations to do *more* with our time? Instead of walking to our coworker to ask a question, we can send an email. Instead of going into our kids' bedroom, we can send them a text. And since body language makes up roughly 55 percent of communication and tone of voice is 38 percent,[52] something always gets lost in translation. What's quickest is not always best, and doing more is not always productive. Shortcuts can lead us into dead ends.

And that's the irony. "Doing more" in our modern workspace usually means doing more things digitally—responding to more emails, messages, and written work. But we know that our bodies suffer for the incongruity of separating work into more mind-engaging and less physically-demanding tasks. When our minds move without our bodies, we feel disconnected. A writer that I follow recently co-wrote a book about how writing has been hurting her body. Another wellness guru is constantly coming up with new biohacks to merge the need for an online digital presence while training for Ironman races. I find that even the experts in the fitness field struggle with our sedentary way of making a living, because the way we make our money is affecting our bodies, our minds, our selves.

I entered the field of corporate wellness after interviewing countless gym members who said they joined because they were active in high school and college, then put on the pounds after having to sit for commutes and at desks in the workplace. A 2018 study in the *Journal of Occupational and Environmental Medicine*[53] reveals how excess weight affects performance: obese workers surveyed were 55 percent more likely to take sick days, and 30 percent were less productive than than their lighter counterparts. It's a catch-22: the traditional workplace environment may cause weight gain, but weight gain is a liability for productivity.

I was a trainer for the Java Gym at Starbucks Corporate and helped employees get an energy boost from thirty-minute lunchtime "Expresso" workouts, fueled by in-house espressos. And for many of them, their short-cuts included fitting in the highest intensity workout in the quickest amount of time. Most were bright-eyed, industrious employees, but some experienced injury and burnout from going too hard, too fast. At another location, I was available as a personal trainer for free, but only about 1 percent of the employees took advantage of this corporate wellness benefit. It may have cost no money, but it cost them joy. They didn't have substantial time during their lunch hour to exercise, and most wanted to clock out and go home, get a break, and not spend any more time at the workplace. Working out at work can feel like more work, instead of a joyful get-to. Companies may want their employees to be healthy and know that exercise increases productivity, but they have a hard time motivating people to participate on-site. Maybe in-house espresso could help.

Exercise doesn't have to be an additional task tacked on to the already packed work day, but woven throughout as an integral part of the process. Since exercise improves cognitive function for complex tasks, executives could encourage employees to exercise before completing a complex task to improve the end result. They could offer stretching videos to follow before engaging in any type of learning endeavor, since it not only improves blood flow and alertness, but elongates the nervous system and opens up synaptic junctions for increased retention. In schools, recess improves test scores. Recess for the workplace, an allotted time for exercise, should be as mandatory to worker's rights as a lunch hour.

Exercise doesn't only benefit jobs outside the home. For the women doing the hard work of creating the next generation, not exercising has consequences for both mamas and babies.

Pregnant moms who lead unhealthy lifestyles may experience excessive weight gain, pre-eclampsia, gestational diabetes, caesarean section, lower back pain, and urinary incontinence.[54] And babies born with a high birth weight are more likely to become obese as children.[55] What we do for our kids in and beyond the womb impacts not only the foundation of their physical makeup, but the formation of the ideas and practices of normal physical activity. Since more adults are sedentary during the day and stay-at-home parents generally exercise less when they become parents, kids are moving less, too. But it's not just the *lack* of exercise that causes our energy slumps and lost work time, but *over exercising* can also bring disastrous results. Let's get to the root of what we need for the day, and include necessary physical activity into our current responsibilities.

Do "time savers" ever take time away from what you really want to do? How?

_____

_____

_____

_____

_____

_____

_____

Write down the time of day you feel least energized. What
are your general habits? Can exercise help?

_____

_____

_____

_____

_____

_____

_____

_____

Another Way

We give so much of ourselves away, whether that is to our business or our family. When do we get filled back up? Parents don't
always get the option of sleeping more at night, but we can make
a way to move during the day. Rest doesn't always have to be
sleep—it can come through exercise too. And if we can find a way
to look forward to it with clear rewards in mind, that excitement
will automatically boost energy levels. The top three excuses
for not exercising are not having enough time, being too tired,
and not getting a break from the kids. But since the Hero is a
life hack aficionado, she can combine the three and arrange to
exercise during her "tired" hours.

Normal energy levels coincide with the amount of cortisol,
or stress hormone, in the body. Usually, cortisol peaks around
8 a.m. and gradually decreases throughout the day to help us
ease into sleep at night, like a slow-release energy pill. Whenever
you feel your cortisol levels dropping along with your eyelids,

consider heading outside for a walk, even if you don't have time. It will boost your energy and make the time you do have more productive. Walking, whether inside or outside, will charge up your battery even when you're tired. And if you have kids, you can walk around inside or close to the house during the afternoon siesta hour. Every step counts!

Clearing Hero Hurdles

Poor planning and life interruptions aren't always the main villains in the Hero's life. Every Hero has her own set of hurdles that will continue to pop up in her path to joy.

Highlight which hurdles you identify with, and learn how you can bounce over them like the energizer bunny you are.

Hurdle #1:

> **Feeling too exhausted from exercise. When sitting becomes controlled falling and your arms can barely lift a fork to your mouth, let alone pick up a needy child, you might have overdone it. You either do something beyond your current level because you're too excited to exercise and skip the warm-up, or too impatient to go through the gradual process of progression .**

Bounce for Joy: Determine your daily needs. Practicing mindfulness will help cue you in to each movement during your exercise routine to determine if it is the right amount for you, for the day, and for your energy levels. Be thankful for the body's simple signals to stop to eat and sleep, and use them to train yourself to know how much energy you'll need from fitness. Think about your Joy Goal before and during the workout to keep yourself "ready for every good work," (2 Timothy 2:21) and adapt your level of activity accordingly.

While stretching and contracting your body, tune in to the sensations of your muscles, joints, and breath all moving together. Turn off the music or any other distractions if needed to do this and get in the zone. Once you get in a regular rhythm of safe movement, distractions can be helpful, but don't skip this initial greeting. Every day is different for your body, so a sufficient warm-up to assess your ability and prepare your body is important every time. If you still feel too sore after a workout, decrease your weight load the next time with a perceived exertion scale. On a threshold of 1-10, if you push yourself above a level 7 (can no longer sing or hold a conversation) keep the intervals short and take sufficient breaks. If you feel bone-tired afterward, lower the intensity or take a few days for restorative movement. Learn more about this method of intuitive training in Chapter Nine.

Be aware that the benefits of exercise taper off after ninety minutes. Prolonged levels of stress, even good stress like exercise, can trigger the breakdown of muscle tissue and suppress the immune system in an effort to bring the body back to homeostasis. Neglecting to rest in between periods of exertion also raises your risk of injury and infection. Give yourself forty-eight hours of rest between strength sessions to allow your systems to rebuild. Rest includes getting enough calories and sleep. If you are unable to get an adequate amount of each, choose a gentle routine until you are in a balanced and stronger state. You will find joy when your workout fills you up and makes you stronger for your greater goals.

Hurdle #2:

> **Loneliness. You want to get everything done, but that means you'll need to do exercise on your own time, and it can feel isolating and unfulfilling, dragging motivation down with the mood.**

Bounce for Joy: *Find a friend.* Every Hero needs a sidekick!

You can still make others a priority without sacrificing your priorities. If you can't work out at the same time as a good friend, start making friends with those who go to the gym or class at the same time as you. If you can only work out at home or can't find a running buddy, invite others to be your workout buddies by checking in through a messaging app or virtual fitness challenge. Set up a time each week to discuss what was fun, what was hard, and ask them for tips. Talking about your struggles with others will help bond you together, increase your joy, and normalize the hardships of fitness to remind you that it's an everyday part of life.

Hurdle #3:

> **Fitness becomes another item on the to-do list.**
> **When your workout becomes another task**
> **item, it can feel like a job instead of a joy.**

Bounce for Joy: *Focus on fun.* When fitness starts feeling more like another thing you feel obligated to do, consider taking a break from your regular routine, and either take some time to rest, or do something that feels like pure fun to restore your joy. If being productive *is* fun for you, start thinking of your to-do list as a to-love list. The Hero is motivated by helping others, so think about whom you are loving as you get stronger through your workout.

Hurdle #4:

> **Lack of focus leads to analysis paralysis**
> **so you don't do anything.**

Bounce for Joy: *Stick to your mission.* As a lifeguard is assigned to a certain portion of the pool, you too are called to stick to your corner. Review your Joy Goal and pray through the Lord's plans for you that day. A good question to ask yourself is, "What is mine to do?" Own it, and train according to your focused assignment. For those times when it feels like you have no time or mental space to think, build a training toolbox. Have two or three workouts that fuel your mission written down so you can refer to them on a minute's notice.

Hurdle #5:

> **Not having enough time or resources. You have good intentions to work out, but the combined feelings of tiredness, and not having enough time to take care of your family (including yourself) leads you to choose other activities over exercise.**

Bounce for Joy: *Stack your life.* Instead of channeling Elastigirl and stretching yourself thin, combine your responsibilities. Since you're the multitasking type, exercise with the people you love. If you have littles, prepare to spend about an hour at at time walking to get the alignment benefits that come with sufficient ambulatory practice. If the kid can walk on her own, walk at her pace. As with any exercise training, kids have to be trained to walk for longer distances. You may not believe highly distractible kids can stay focused, but my mind was changed after I jogged my three-year-old in a stroller a 5K. We were right behind a child smaller than mine who held hands and ran with his mom for 1.5 miles straight. That little boy made me a believer in the long-distance ability of youngsters! To keep kids on track, pick a narrow path. It has less distractions and will naturally lead them forward.

You can pick a time when you need the most energy or when everyone can do it together. Since walking is a low-intensity exercise, you can even do this later in the day after dinner to aid digestion and enhance sleep (and what parent wouldn't do anything for more sleep?) instead of plopping in front of a screen, which has blue light and flashing signals that can interfere with how your brain transitions into rest.

You can actually over-wire your brain with artificially stimulating substances like caffeine, sugar, television, and video games so they become like drugs, and you constantly need more to feel the same rush of pleasure.[56] Replace these with more natural hits of epinephrine and dopamine through exercise, sunshine, and spending time in nature. Studies on forest bathing (meditatively strolling through the woods) have been proven to be more mentally restorative and stimulating than watching a show on television.

Jesus is the Hero

One of the biggest joy hurdles for the Hero is when exercise feels like a necessary inconvenience. A joyless exercise routine won't last when life gets hard. The Hero needs to find her strength not in what she does, but who she is in Christ and who He is in her. Only then can she endure for the long-run!

When there's too much to do and she doesn't have support, the Hero can identify with the Samaritan woman at the well in John 4. Working out can feel like having to go to the well for water, in the blazing heat, day after day. But instead of us spending ourselves, Jesus meets us there and offers us something that will never run out: "If you knew the gift of God, and who it is that is saying to you, 'Give me a drink,' you would have asked him, and he would have given you living water" (John 4:10). And like the woman, we may think, "Wonderful! Does that mean I can do this once and be good to go for life?"

Well, no. Jesus isn't saying that we don't need water, that we don't need exercise. He demonstrated this by asking for water *after* He had just commuted on foot. Jesus demonstrates His needs to show us ours. The woman needed water, but her obstacle was shame.

What is our biggest obstacle to exercise? At my 2 p.m. slump,

I needed energy, but my obstacle was fear of not getting it all done. And if I didn't get it all done, I wasn't doing enough, and perhaps I thought that *I* wasn't enough. I was looking to my accomplishments to save myself. But when they invent that magic exercise pill I won't have to worry about taking time away from my agenda anymore. I had the mindset of the women at the well: "When the Messiah comes, he'll explain everything" (John 4:25).

But right when we've admitted our need for a Higher Power bigger than our obstacles, Jesus pulls off the Messiah mask and shows us that what we hope for is right in front of us: "I, the one speaking to you—I am he" (John 4:26). *Gasp* The big reveal! The beggar is actually the big hero!

This story shows I don't have to keep digging in the well of fitness (or lack thereof) for the saving answer. I don't have to keep staring at the obstacles that keep coming up, but trust in the One who is already there. My Savior, my hero, is Jesus! And as the woman leaves her water jar and runs back to face the people she feared, we can leave our ways of striving to do more and to do it better. He has already done it! The smartest thing the Hero can do is to walk in the truth that the work of salvation is finished.

If you need energy today, what is stopping you from using movement like a bucket into the well?

_____

_____

_____

_____

_____

"If only you knew the gift of God...and who it is....you would ask him" (John 4):

Instead of asking exercise what you want out of it, imagine Jesus saying to you, I, the one speaking to you—I am he" (John 4:26). As you picture yourself putting down your leaky jar of striving, breathe a deep sigh of relief, and let your shoulders relax from the weight of carrying the tension of bearing it all. As you inhale, imagine Jesus' living water filling your lungs. Do you feel more energized in mind, body, and/or spirit?

The woman at the well went back to her people to tell the good news of the Savior. Who do you need to share this with?

_____

_____

_____

What the Hero Wants

The ultimate desire for the Hero is letting Jesus be the hero within.

Exercise fills you with Kingdom power.

Common sense says that a vessel needs to be full to be poured out. But when we are focused on our own agenda, even when that includes having a "fit" body, we never feel satisfied. Dissatisfaction is a sign of a leaky vessel. To fill ourselves up, we may use exercise as a distraction from our problems, or avoid it because it seems too time-consuming.

After the woman at the well left, Jesus' friends showed up and asked if He wanted to get a bite to eat. He mysteriously answered (with a wink to the readers) that He was already full. Doing the work of the Lord, though it may empty us of what we think we want, fills us up with what we need. Jesus is the ultimate time-Savior! He doesn't give us more hours in the day, He redeems the activities of our day. Exercise may feel like it empties us of our energy, but it actually gives us more. This mystery is a taste of Kingdom accomplishment. As we become less, He becomes greater! As we empty ourselves in service of the Lord, His presence patches the holes, makes us whole, and we overflow with joy.

My friend Sarah took advantage of a chunk free time to do just that. She explains how He multiplied her one hour into more for her week:

> *All my kiddos were taken care of this morning, and I got out for a little early morning soul care. I mostly hiked with a little running here and there. The point wasn't doing it at a certain pace or in a particular time. I love it. I enjoyed a good podcast, on a book I'm actually reading as part of a book club, which has really changed my ideas on rest in the best ways. Then I listened to worship music from one of my playlists. Worship music is my jam. I may not have gotten much sleep last night, but I feel so much more ready to tackle my week after this morning.*

Her walk with the Lord energized her for the rest of the day! The Hero wants to be a whole and holy vessel, ready to refresh others with the Lord's strength. Like Sarah, we must fix our eyes and focus on God's work in order to be fit for service.

The Hero's Core Verse

Let's dig deeper into the well with the Hero's verse, and draw out a drink one section at a time:

> *"Therefore, if anyone cleanses himself from what is dishonorable, he will be a vessel for honorable use, set apart as holy, useful to the master of the house, ready for every good work."*
>
> 2 TIMOTHY 2:21

If anyone cleanses himself from what is dishonorable: The word "cleanse" means to purge, or clean out. As we regularly put vessels, like water bottles, into the dishwasher to be clean to drink from, how are we cleansing the vessel of our bodies? Our body is naturally efficient at cleansing itself from toxins without any help. Sweat can expedite the process, but it takes a little work on our part.

While sweat rids us of our toxins, it can also purge the built-up gunk of pride. Sweating is a sign of exertion, and can feel vulnerable. One barrier I came across while working in the corporate wellness world was that higher-up executives typically avoided working out with their employees. I assumed one of the reasons was because sweating can be a sign of weakness. It was important to maintain their position of authority both in the gym and the workplace.

Pushing yourself to the point of sweat, just like giving yourself permission to cry, or standing out in the pouring rain, is a baptism of sorts. It's a public proclamation that says, "I'm letting go," training you to release the pride in other areas of your life that hold you back from your God-given purpose. For me, this means ordering groceries online, or asking for more help around the house, so I can get in a workout and feel more focused and joyful for what I'm called to do.

What do you need to clean from your life that is not from the Lord?

_____

_____

_____

_____

_____

What busy tasks clog up your schedule and wear you out?

_____

_____

_____

_____

_____

Where do you need to put down your pride and pick up a barbell?

_____

_____

_____

_____

He will be a vessel for honorable use, set apart as holy: This word "honorable" refers to being of value in the eyes of the beholder.

Who is your beholder or the person for whom you want to be useful?

_____

_____

_____

How can you be set apart for special use instead of follow-ing along with the rat race? This can look like stepping outside during lunch hour while everyone else is eating indoors, or modifying an exercise to show honor to your body (and its Maker) instead of competing with everyone else in the class.

_____

_____

_____

_____

Useful to the master of the house: Think of something that has collected dust in your house—is it your Bible, the treadmill, or yoga mat? What we do not use gets buried and eventually deteriorates over time. Make it a daily practice to shake off the dust and move from head to toe, feeling the joy flow through every part of your body.

Ready for every good work: When we make ourselves useful, we can be ready for every good work, defined as an action completing an inner desire. When my mom taught my sister and me to play tennis, she constantly had to tell me, "Stay on your toes!" because I would stand on the other side of the court, flat-footed. Twenty years later, I hear the same thing from my boxing instructor. And this time, I listen, because if I don't, I will miss ducking a punch and get socked right in the face. Mom, I wouldn't have blamed you if you hit me with the ball just to teach my stubborn self a lesson! Being ready for every good work is keeping your eyes on the Master and staying on your toes, keeping your body moving and ready to spring for joy.

Joy Gifts of the Hero

A Hero always uses his superpowers to help someone else, to make the world a better place. And in doing so, he is fulfilled. When your superpowers come from the Lord, they never run out. Making the world a better place in the Lord means bringing eternal heaven on Earth, one assignment at a time. Here are your joy gifts to have and to share:

- **You are full of energy:** Others might marvel at how much energy you have to work and work out. You know that exercise aids digestion to absorb more nutrients, decreases PMS symptoms, chronic pain, sparks creativity, and increases sleep quality to help you feel more energized during the day. "In the poll of 1,000 people, those who exercised the most vigorously reported the best sleep quality overall. And they were less likely than non-exercisers to say that in the past two weeks, they had experienced problems such as trouble falling asleep or waking during the night."[57]

Share this gift by engaging in activities that not only burn off the extra energy, but fill you back up with the joy that you so readily give to others.

- **You are thirsty to serve:** You are like an eager waiter with your eyes on the empty cups at the tables assigned to you, ready to fill them up at a moment's notice.

Enhance this joy gift by combining physical activity with community service, such as volunteering with Habitat for Humanity, running for charities, or starting up your own neighborhood prayer walks. You can even do this in exercise classes, like setting up equipment for others or helping the instructor with activities.

The Hero can stop trying to save everyone around her to feel saved. She is allowed (nay, encouraged!) to spend time doing what fills her up with joy. Making time for activities that fill her up give her the energy she needs for her Joy Goal.

Exercise

If the Hero wants to fly, she has to be grounded. She needs to know where she comes from, she needs to be oriented with the earth beneath her feet so she doesn't fly too close to the sun. Katy Bowman says that the most unused exercise equipment is the floor.[58] Most of us don't get on the floor because we have furniture that acts as a shortcut on the way down. Yes, the floor can be dirty—but you know what that means—bonus movement to get down and get it clean! Getting all the way down and up from the ground is a full body movement. If we remember 10 percent of what we read, 20 percent of what we hear, 30 percent of what we see, 50 percent of what we see and hear, 70 percent of what we say and write, 80 percent of what we experience, and 90 percent of what we say and do, let us say, "The joy of the Lord is my strength" while we do this exercise.[59]

Practice digging deep into the well of humility by lowering yourself so you are face down on the ground and rise to standing. Repeat five to six times a day. You can even pretend that you have no furniture in your house and sit on the floor as a regular practice.

Put Your Cape On

Two o'clock in the afternoon is still a struggle, but I no longer feel stuck on the high-carb path for energy and productivity. I realized that it was a problem for me, and awareness is the first step to change. Going outside, even if it's just to walk two houses down and back, gives me the boost of circulation and sunshine I need. I can even answer email on my phone while I go! But I've found that I am better when I can set aside focused time for each task and not try to mash everything together. I have started enjoying the walks and drag my daughter along when I can.

Now, she is the one who begs me to race down the massive hill right outside our front door. One time before we went out, I was showing her my new illustrated anatomy book, and she pointed to the hip bones and said, "Butterfly wings!" I always thought our wings would sprout from our shoulder blades, and that we had to imagine ourselves flying (or put on a special red cape), but she saw something I did not. God already gave us wings! As I ran beside her, watching her fly down that hill with wind whipping through her hair, my own lungs emptied and my heart filled up.

Hero Quick Reference Guide

When you need to remember what gets you going, refer to the statements below:

Hero motivation: Enjoying the Lord through exercise equips you for every good work.

Joy declaration: I will move for joy and be filled with energy to advance the Kingdom.

Hero prayers to be used for exercise:
- "As I move my body, may You move me."
- "Sow energy, reap energy."
- "Fill me with Your presence."

If you are a Hero and are ready to get going, skip to Chapter Eight to start planning your Joy Goal.

Chapter Six

The Warrior: Do Something Awesome

I had never worked so hard in a spin class. When my corporate wellness boss signed the whole team of personal trainers up for a group bonding exercise at spin class, my competitive side came out. Yes, I needed to impress her with my physical abilities, but I also needed to hold my own amongst my peers.

We entered the gym, where the staff asked what we wanted our screen names to be. They would track our effort based on our bike number's imported stats, and post our scores through our screen name on a board for all to see. This was completely optional, but I like a good challenge, so I accepted. After we got strapped in, the lights got low and the music turned up. It was officially game time. We pedaled to the beat as the spin instructor encouraged us to reach our "better" while I glanced at one of the company's hashtags, #nevercoast. I narrowed my eyes, powered up my legs, and got into the groove.

Then I saw my name on the board! But every time I started to decrease my tempo, my name dropped down the list. I was tired, but I was motivated by competition. I kicked up the resistance on my bike to add more points. One of my coworkers was killing it, the other opted out of the public stats display, and then my goal turned into: "Stay on the board. Don't. Be. Last." The tenets of success for this particular gym, along with others like it, are achievement, purpose, and belonging—three factors that play into the essence of the Warrior.

Why We Need to Be the Warrior

Fitness can often feel arbitrary. We feel the sweat, but we need someone to tell us exactly how many calories we have burned so we can do better next time. By assigning point values, fitness feels more like a fun game with goals to reach and less like an endless treadmill to nowhere. The new challenges presented at each workout feel like a different mountaintop to summit, and you leave feeling like a conqueror. As a result of these small victories, you're more equipped to battle conflict at work, deal with the stress of moving to another house, and weather relational storms. Exercising strengthens the Warrior for life's struggles.

When we are empowered within, we feel confident to branch out. We are created with a desire to enjoy all of God's creation, which often starts with discovering all of what our own bodies can do: "No man has the right to be an amateur in the matter of physical training. It is a shame for a man to grow old without seeing the beauty and strength of which his body is capable." [60] Competition plays a key role in unleashing what we are each capable of. Ecclesiastes says that "all toil and achievement spring from one person's envy of another."[61] It's not just in humans, but in cockroaches, too!

While they are still my household nemesis, in this case they teach me a valuable lesson. In one study, researchers directed roaches to run on a straight track, and when they put cockroaches in the makeshift stands, the roaches did better. However, when the roaches were directed with light to make more difficult turns on a track with the audience, they fared worse.[62] Our behavior clearly changes when others watch us.[63] We can attribute our awareness *of* others to the need to survive *with* others—after all, the joy response is linked to the collective effort rather than attending to individual needs.

History proves that people together are stronger than one person alone. Ancient cultures like the Assyrians, Babylonians, and Egyptians trained their young men to be soldiers to protect their country through defense and conquest. Greeks created the Olympics with events that mimicked war skills, such as running, the javelin toss, jumping, striking, and wrestling. After World Wars I and II, Americans were more motivated by recreational activities than training for potential military threats. Dwight D. Eisenhower established the President's Council on Youth Fitness in 1956 to raise up generations of health-conscious Americans, and John F. Kennedy published "The Soft American" in Sports Illustrated to address the country's unhealthy body compositions. With the rise of technology, we need our bodies less for physical combat. However, survival is still on the line, albeit on a different scale.

In a 2016 interview with *Politico,* U.S. Surgeon General Dr. Vivek Murthy said the most common illness today isn't heart disease, diabetes, or cancer (the top three reported leading causes of death). The top threat is to our health is...

Social isolation. Dr. Murthy went on to say: "...we underestimate how prevalent isolation is. We underestimate the impact it has on our health. In fact, we know that social isolation–science tells us, in fact–that social isolation is linked to shorter lives, to cognitive decline, to increased rates of cardiovascular disease, as well as other healthcare concerns."[64] And for the record, social media does not count as socializing when it comes meeting our holistic needs. Behind our screens, we are alone together. But one of the joy chemicals, oxytocin, the one that gives us a warm and fuzzy feeling as a reward for fulfilling the essential need for human bonding, is only released when we are physically present with one another.

When we combine togetherness with fitness, we gain consistency in our health habits. One study paired participants in a weight-loss program with three friends and compared their results with those who tried to do the program alone. Ninety-five percent of those who did the program with friends completed it, compared to only a 76 percent completion rate for the solitary participants. The friends group was also 42 percent more likely to maintain their weight loss after the four and ten month check-ins.[65]

Restoring Joy by Removing Comparison

While friendly competition is beneficial, it can be detrimental to our bodies and lead us off course. We may try and go beyond our level of fitness to fit in with the rest of the class and get injured. We may become discouraged when we don't score enough points, get jealous of someone else's performance, or feel unwanted when the regulars don't invite us to hang out after class. It can feel like a personal assault on our ability and identity, blocking our joy.

Josh from Alabama shares his story of how God has restored joy in movement by removing comparison:

> *Even though I am a group fitness trainer, for years I have struggled with insecurities about my place and contribution in the fitness community. There are a lot of comparisons, a lot of striving, making sure you're lifting more than someone else. I often felt like I wasn't good enough, strong enough, or equipped to lead others in movement. However, in the fall of 2017, I walked through a new fitness certification called Revelation Wellness, a faith-based fitness ministry. They kept saying things like: 'You be you. Be who God created you to be. Don't be more than that and know that God has great things in store for you.' Instead of focusing on what I was not, I am free to walk in my original design and bless others. I can wholly enjoy my duty of making my body a healthy temple and lead others into God's reckless love to reclaim movement for themselves, too.*

The Last Will Be First

Josh's story is not unusual. Even the twelve disciples were not immune to striving for the best spot amongst each other. At the Passover feast when Jesus shares the bread and wine as His body and blood of the new covenant, He declares that He must be given over in betrayal. But woe to the one who gives Him over! The disciples immediately start questioning each other of who Jesus could be talking about, trying to figure out who is the worst among them and making sure it wasn't them.

This conversation of who was the worst promptly lead into a dispute over who was the best in the very next verse. Jesus overhead their argument and settled it fair and square: whoever was the winner of an extreme discipleship obstacle course would be crowned the winner (complete with yeast quicksand traps and Pharisee stumbling stones). Or at least that's how I would have done it. But Jesus is God and He's way better than me, so He set up a different kind of competition: "let the greatest among you become as the youngest, and the leader as one who serves" (Luke 22:26). And while they were arguing over who was the best, while Peter boasted about how He would follow Him anywhere, Jesus was getting crucified. All deserted Him.

The Warrior feels this pain of loneliness when she makes plans to workout with a friend who stands her up, or plans an exercise class and nobody shows. The weight of an empty room is crushing. The Warrior feels the ache of rejection and yet still puts herself out there because she longs for connection. Even when nobody is willing to run beside her, even if nobody comes, Jesus always does. He is always right beside you.

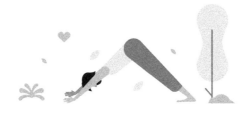

The Warrior's Core Verse

Athletes are often compared to warriors—they are not distracted by the ways of the world but keep their eyes on the prize:

> *"Watching [athletes], we are inspired to test the limits of our own bodies and our own lives. No wonder the apostle Paul so often draws on the image of the athlete to inspire new Christians to embrace their path with rigor, singleness of purpose, self-control, perseverance, and endurance. No wonder the prophets used images of physical strength to describe the coming reign of God."*
> STEPHANIE PAULSELL[66]

The Warrior works out to build up the body of Christ. The Warrior suffers most when he is alone and underchallenged. To find joy in fitness, he needs to focus on pursuing a goal with others. Getting together with others releases oxytocin, doing something rewarding releases dopamine, and he gets a boost of adrenaline by taking a risk.

To connect his fitness habits with the source of joy, he will need to add these fighting words of Scripture to his arsenal.:

> *"Instead, speaking the truth in love, we will grow to become in every respect the mature body of him who is the head, that is, Christ. From him the whole body, joined and held together by every supporting ligament, grows and builds itself up in love, as each part does its work."*
> EPHESIANS 4:15-16

Instead, speaking the truth in love: The root of "speaking the truth" literally translates to "truthing," or making a record of what God deems is truth rather than personal illusion.[67]

When you hit a personal best or break a record, what is your first response? Is it to broadcast it to the world, or to give praise to the One who gifted you, empowered you, and was with you through the finish line?

_____

_____

_____

_____

_____

What about when you fail? Do you blame it on a trainer, on a vacation, or do you stand strong and preach to yourself, "His power is made perfect in my weakness"?[68]

_____

_____

_____

_____

_____

How you respond to fitness victories and failures speak volumes about who you worship and what you believe. The Warrior speaks the truth in love for the joy of all who hear.

We will grow to become in every respect the mature body of him who is the head, that is, Christ: The Olympic motto is, "*Citius,*

Altius, Fortius." Faster, Higher, Stronger. You may not dream of being an Olympic athlete, but we all want better for ourselves. We see kids one-upping each other on the playground, college students comparing each other's top fitness tracker scores, and the fitness industry training its clients like professional athletes.

But is it a realistic goal to expect ourselves to get continuously fitter over time, even as we age? The following factors as told on the TED Talks stage by David Epstein indicate we are not done with athletic improvement: "innovation in sports, whether that's new track surfaces or new swimming techniques, the democratization of sport, the spread to new bodies and to new populations around the world, and imagination in sport, an understanding of what the human body is truly capable of, have conspired to make athletes stronger, faster, bolder, and better than ever."[69]

Bret Stetka, the author of an article titled, "Have We Reached the Athletic Limits of the Human Body," sides with the laws of physics that humanity as a whole can't keep this up for long, unless we change the rules ourselves: "I think people will find ways to enhance oxygen delivery through the body and squeeze more performance out of humans. The only question is will these approaches be considered legal."[70]

As we know, the human body's improvements are bound by physics. However, God has "immeasurably more" in store for us, and the Warrior's joy is in pursuing the more! Challenging our physical limits, whatever they may be in life, is a picture of how to unleash spiritual growth.

Try and do push-ups until you can't. In the process of finding your limit, you'll grow past it. Doing push-ups until failure ultimately strengthens your muscles. The joy of fitness is to discover our limits by pushing past them.

Jesus is always calling us upward and onward. He will always have a new challenge for us, but it will never be for our own glory. There are no rogue soldiers in the Kingdom. Just as cancer is a cell that has gone its own way, we become destructive when we work (or work out) to establish ourselves. As the saying goes, "Alone we can go fast, but together we can go far." Let us reach the far-off finish line together under Jesus's headship, finding joy by playing within the uniting framework of the body.

From him the whole body, joined and held together by every supporting ligament: While the Warrior can feel alone if she's not with someone, she is always connected to others. The Warrior already has two essential points of contact:

1. *Structure:* Physical contact with others as a muscle is connected to a bone.
2. *Power:* Spiritual contact with the Lord as a muscle's nerve endings connect to the brain.

The muscles, bones, and connective tissue give the body structure, but the nerve impulses from the brain make it move. When the body's parts are disconnected from the signals of the brain, it leads into what is called kinesthetic dysfunction, which is "a problem with how you perceive the messages coming from your kinesthetic receptors. You need two things to correct kinesthetic dysfunction: new sensory input and a willingness to pay attention to it."[71] The brain-body connection is not always automatic, nor is the spiritual walk without work. Quickly practice this concept by looking at your pinky toe and telling only it to move, while keeping the other toes still. This new challenge creates awareness and submission to the central nervous system commands. It is a pattern of the relationship between the two points of contact.

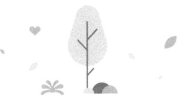

Did your pinky toe listen to you? How often are you submitting to the Lord's directions for your movements, as your body listens to your commands? Draw one line to connect the circles for "rarely," two lines for "sometimes" and three lines for "quick to submit."

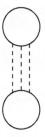

Your pinky toe is automatically connected to your other body parts, just as we are connected to each other, but we don't often do you acknowledge and appreciate the other members of the body. How well are you connecting with others in your fitness ambitions? Draw one line to connect the circles for "not so well," two lines for "getting by" and three lines to symbolize a "strong connection."

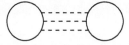

What is a new challenge you can engage in to strengthen these connections and increase joy?

_____

_____

_____

_____

...grows and builds itself up in love, as each part does its work: As a football team can only successfully get the ball across the field through the cooperation of a quarterback, a tight end, a lineman, etc., so we each have a position to play. There is no room for comparison in the body of Christ. Know your part, and build up one another in love with training tips, affirmation, and encouragement. If you are not sure of your part, continue to Chapter Eight to discover your design.

Conquering Hurdles

When drawing up a battle plan, all enemy obstacles must be identified. Know yours and move forward in Christ, becoming more than a conqueror.

Hurdle #1:

> *Lack of a plan. If you don't have a goal, a race date, or a team to show up for, you tend to fall off the wayside.*

Conquer for joy: *Get a goal.* Find out what you need, what brings you joy, and pick a realistic and fitting activity. You will flesh this out in Chapters Eight and Nine. Take one action step toward it today, even if that simply means reading the rest of this chapter.

Hurdle #2:

> *Inconsistency. If you don't have somebody working out with you or something to show up for, you find it hard to keep up a regular schedule.*

Conquer for joy: *Reach out.* Warriors need to know there are other soldiers battling with them in the trenches of life. We are far more likely to stick with an exercise regimen when others are dependent upon our participation, even if it's not a team effort. Consider the standard yoga or Pilates class. Each involves individual-based tasks that require you to work alone in the presence of others. You may be able to focus better by yourself, but you'll show up more consistently and gain more creative inspiration by surrounding yourself with others. There's even a term for the euphoric social bonding that occurs when humans get together and start moving: *collective effervescence.*

If you want to increase that bubbly joy, research suggests that simply working out in the same space is not nearly as effective as exercising as being part of a team. Any activity that focuses on your increasing competence contributing to a team's success, and your failure to show impacting everyone, levels up the possibility of you coming, getting better, and having more fun.[72]

If you're not ready to jump into a team sport or learn a new skill, consider investing in a gym or competition ahead of time. Make sure it's the right fit for you and your Joy Goal, then decide how much you want to pay in advance. You might not have friends there at first, but you'll be motivated to get your money's worth and make friends on the way. A few more tips for connecting your fitness journey with others:

- Practice inviting the Lord in. You're never alone, and He's always enough.
- Think of those in your own house: they are your tribe, and children are your quiver of arrows. Raise up that army!
- Outside of the family, seek out a training partner, sign up for a team, or head to a challenging group fitness class.

Hurdle #3:

No visible results. If you aren't seeing growth or get injured, you tend to get discouraged.

Conquer for Joy: *Focus on learning.* Instead of recording failures, count every opportunity as a challenge to learn something new. Get hurt? Become the best at recovering. Aren't experiencing forward progress? Focus on the process, how you feel, and what you could do differently. Bring out the conqueror in you and meet your challenges head-on.

If you're getting frustrated in a plateau, add variety to allow your body to work in a different way. Then, invite someone else in who is slightly above your level to challenge you. One study shows that those who planked with a more experienced partner increased their plank time by 24 percent.[73] The goal is never to reach a certain number, but to exalt God's name by using every resource He has given you, which includes using your creativity and sometimes enlisting a team of support to overcome an obstacle. Just being around others can double the fun, and the effort! Human beings naturally want to sync with one another, and one way the body does that is through the heart. The heart's electrical field, which can reach eight to ten feet away, can have an emotional impact on anyone within proximity. This means you can feed off of your exercise partner's positivity simply by being with them!

Hurdle #4

Competing with a more "in shape" version of yourself.

Conquer for Joy: *Know your season.* The Scriptures that declare you as a new creation in Christ and that God's mercies are new every morning have scientific backing as well. The body's cells are constantly turning over (admittingly at different rates, so the myth that you get a new body every seven years doesn't technically apply) and being replaced by new cells. The body you have today literally is not the body you had yesterday. Greet your body as brand new each day, not expecting it to perform or look like it did yesterday (and especially not like it did when you were in high school). What hurt last week may be better today, or what worked to make you faster last year might not jive with your current life demands.

To discover what your abilities are for each workout, try testing your mobility beforehand with the same warm-up exercises. Doing this will bring awareness to present limitations and newfound range of motion freedoms. Knowing your body intimately will help you train more intuitively, empowering you to do what is best for you and not try to meet expectations of your past, a present program, or a future version of yourself. Joy is not a static state but a flowing, fluid strength empowered by God's renewing Spirit. It's worth taking the time and energy to discern what that joy looks like for you today. You can find more on intuitive training in Chapter Nine.

Hurdle #5:

Needing to prove yourself to others by what you can do.

Conquer for Joy: *Fight the right fight. Fight the good fight.* While it may feel good to perform well in front of others (like I wanted to for my boss and coworkers on the spin bike), this feeling does not sit upon a firm foundation. It only feeds pride. Pride puffs up, while maturity builds up. We gain nothing in the long run by being faster, better, or stronger than someone else. And to get down to the heart of it, let me say that your worth is not in how well you do, but in what Jesus has done. Jesus had no need to prove to anyone that He was God by performing the miracles that others demanded. Jesus knew how much His Father loved Him, Jesus knew the path set for Him, and Jesus knew the victory crown laid up for Him at the end. That's someone I want to partner with for my race!

The Greek word used for *athlete* in the Bible means "to contend, to wrestle." We will struggle to remember that God may not keep a record of our physical feats in themselves because

He does not focus on the outward appearance, but as a woman named Jill reminded me in a wellness challenge, "God does count something…righteousness which comes from faith (our faith is counted as righteousness). God's response is grace which is available to all through Christ Jesus. The same grace is available for a starving man and an obese man. There is no comparison in grace."

So if you want to fight the good fight, it's not to beat someone else, because their race is not yours. Don't get yourself disqualified through distraction from your path or attraction to another's. Fix your eyes on the Lord and finish the race God has given you. He will give you overflowing joy to bless those battling beside you. And since we don't fight each other, we fight *with* each other. Reinforce this truth in your own fitness practice by giving frequent high-fives, shouts of encouragement, and doing celebration dances together during competition. Encouraging one another through these types of physical contact have been shown to increase performance *and* enjoyment.[74]

Joy Gifts of the Warrior

I had this breakthrough with God to just lay down the cynicism and become authentic and be who he has created me to be… I'm blown away by what God still has for me and what He has planned for me. I've learned how to be healthy and how to be loved… He's peeling back things in my heart and life and my past that God has allowed me to go through so I can be something beautiful for someone else. Our wives need us, our sons need us, our daughters need us. They need us to step up to the plate. God has given us a heart for this world. Let's stop hiding in the shadows.
-Nick, Revelation Wellness Instructor[75]

Every soldier is gifted and skilled in different areas. Nick laid out a challenge for the Warrior: stop hiding in the shadows. Use your gifts and fight for the light of joy!

- **Being the best for the rest**: You striving to become the best person God has created you to be inspires and strengthens others. You see "outdo one another in showing honor" (Romans 12:10) as a worthy challenge. You don't let yourself fall for excuses, but push past them for the joy of another. You take Jesus at His word and strive to become the best servant leader.

    Share this joy gift by coaching, mentoring, or training with someone else who needs your spark and skills. Some of the best conversations happen while on the move. Once you feel like they're ready, train them to disciple someone else, building up a salvation army.

- **You don't settle for mediocre:** You are constantly seeking, searching, growing, and improving. God gives you the command: "love others," and you make it your ambition to do it more and more, to lead a peaceful life, working hard with your hands, doing your own part and beyond as God has given it to you.

    Enhance this joy gift by turning your workouts into prayers of sanctification: as you learn perseverance and strength in your training, ask God to use that time to grow you spiritually within the bounds of His grace.

Empowering Others

In that spin class with my coworkers, there were many times my mind said, "I can't!" Maybe it was because I had never exerted that much effort before and I was entering into unknown territory. Maybe it was because I was relying on myself and I didn't believe in my abilities. Maybe it was because my legs were burning and I didn't like that.

Then, I remembered the Lord.

I remembered a time when I was paralyzed with anxiety, and all I could hear was the crushing blow of the belief that "I can't." But a stronger voice responded and said, "You're right. But I can." *That* set me free from myself, relieved me as commander of my own post, and placed me into the ranks of faith where there are no limits. Sure, I can do all things in Christ, but the secret is not just the ability to achieve, but joy in the struggle. And the struggle for me was to let go of competition and to grab on to the victory of the Lord.

I looked up from my own spin bike stats and saw my coworkers not as competition but as fellow workers with me. I loosened my furrowed brow and focused on cheering them on instead. It really helped take the focus off my own pain!

"The only way to successfully compete in this race is to make sure someone else wins it."[76]

We all wobbled away from the bikes, slapped sweaty high fives, took a group picture as proof, and laughed as we sipped our smoothie reward. To this day I don't remember who was first, but I do remember that we did it together.

Chest Press Exercise

For this exercise, all you need is your own two hands. Press your palms together in front of your chest while drawing your shoulder blades together and rolling the heads of your shoulders back. Now press your hands together as tight as you can, as if they are two separate entities vying for the center spot in front of your chest. Keeping the same isometric intensity, start pumping your hands up and down

about one inch. As you do so, your chest gets stronger.
You hands may seem separate, but as they press into one
another, they strengthen the body. Let this be a reminder
to press into one another, building up the whole body of
Christ, together.

Warrior Quick Reference Guide

When you need to remember what gets you going, refer to the
statements below:

Warrior motivation: Enjoying the Lord through exercise is
victory.

Joy Declaration: "I will build up the body of Christ by giving
my best and connecting others to the joy of movement."

Warrior prayers to be used for exercise:
- "After you, Lord!"
- "Let's do this!"
- "His love never quits"

If you are a Warrior, you may skip to Chapter Eight to begin
conquering your Joy Goal plan.

Chapter Seven

The Keeper: Stay Healthy

I feel as though I'm doing things right: abiding by all the pregnancy books' recommendations to eat the right foods and avoid the sushi, exercise regularly, manage my stress, and take time to rest. But my body is still breaking. Blue veins and stretch marks spread across my third-trimester body, like an egg shell ready to hatch. People say to me, "You must be due any day now!" and I respond with, "Yes, I'm only seven weeks away!" and pause for their mixed reactions of shock and embarrassment.

I both feel *and* look like I could have a baby any minute now, but I still have quite some time in this body that seems to be falling apart (right where my hips meet). I have all the baby gear ready, so I could spend the rest of the next two months lying down and relaxing. But I still take short walks when my feet hurt, take my four-year-old to the pool so I can swim too, and I bought a special prenatal Pilates subscription online. Why go through all the trouble when my body is going to practically split open and I'll need to start over after weeks of recovery?

Why Keep Up with Our Dying Bodies?

During pregnancy, I did my best to take care of myself, because when I did, I took care of my baby. I wanted to make her a cozy, healthy home. What makes a house a home? For me, a home is an ordered space filled with framed memories, cozy blankets, a full fridge, and room for family and guests to rest and play. A home is a launching pad for the rest of life. Exercise helps make my body a home by providing regular cleaning through sweat, strengthening myself for others, storing muscle memories, and getting the blood flowing through all parts to make a unified space of peace filled with energy and rest when I need it. When our body is a home we love, we want to take care of it.

Your body is a home, too.

What makes a joyful home for you?

_____

_____

_____

_____

How can exercise make your body a joyful home?

_____

_____

_____

_____

_____

We only have this one home for our whole lives. When we are young, we don't think about it much because everyone around us is relatively healthy. But when we get older, we see more of our friends and family affected by various illnesses and many afflictions that can be prevented by diet and exercise, like diabetes or heart disease. After we hit thirty, our metabolism starts to slow down and we see firsthand the beginning effects of aging, with the extra weight that won't seem to go away like it used to. As the numbers grow on the scale and on the cake, we realize that we aren't getting any younger, and that no one else is responsible for our bodies and health but us.

The Keeper knows we are not renters, but homeowners. And if we don't invest in the home of our body with regular maintenance, we start feeling the consequences. Regular exercise not only maintains health, but lowers rates of high blood pressure, diabetes, and cancer.[77] It also extends the quality of joints, maintains muscle mass, and keeps bones strong to keep us fit to run the race and experience the Keeper's Joy Goal of stewarding her resources well for life. Exercise is an act of thanksgiving for all she has been given.

The Keeper knows we are not the only ones affected by what we do (or don't do) with our bodies. Exercise improves immunity, in effect contributing to herd immunity, the concept that the collective wellness of a people group strengthens overall resistance to disease. How we take care of ourselves directly affects the next generation, and the Keeper is conscious of that. She will find the built-in joy when she listens to the needs of her own body for the health of others. Long-term sustainability for the good of all is central to the Keeper's Joy Goal.

When a woman is pregnant, she may be aware that what she does affects the baby, but new studies show that how the mother takes care of the baby in her womb can affect the baby's genetic composition. The term for this is fetal origins of disease. For example, a baby may carry the gene for diabetes, but lifestyle habits have the power to turn gene on or off. If a mother does not make wise lifestyle, exercise, or nutrition decisions during pregnancy, it can increase the risk of turning on the diabetes gene in both mother and baby.[78] The Keeper is not motivated by fear, but is wise enough to have a healthy fear of the real enemies of malady that can be brought on by our own action (or inaction).

If we have kids, the moment they come in to the world is the point we truly realize our physical inadequacy. Children are more excited to wake up early (maybe because they haven't pulled a muscle while sleeping), run circles around us during the day, and when they fall and scrape their knees, they bounce back up again with the help of a kiss and a bandage. The older we get, the harder it gets to rise from a fall. But we know that exercise can help slow the hands of time to give us more vitality and years with our loved ones.

As we age, the capacity for our cells to divide over and over again decreases. The telltale marker of aging is the length of our telomeres, which are the protective caps on the ends of chromosomes, and they get shorter with each replication. But moderate intensity exercise has been shown to lengthen lifespan by as much as five years! One study[79] monitored ten healthy people before and after a forty-five-minute stationary bike ride. The bout of exercise increased levels of a molecule that helps to protect telomeres, extending their lifespans and essentially the exerciser's life.

For those who haven't been exercising at all, a person's risk of dying prematurely decreased by nearly 20 percent simply by meeting the current exercise guidelines of 150 minutes of moderate activity per week.[80] Muscles are a reservoir, a containment center for anti-aging hormones. People who have more muscle age better, recover faster, and look younger.[81] We want not only to live longer, but feel better aging. The anti-aging market is only projected to grow with time[82] as we seek out solutions for wrinkles and sagging skin. Our monetary investments reflect our desire to *look* younger. The Keeper is not motivated by external appearances, but by general long-term maintenance. The Keeper is eager to please, but if she gets distracted and tries to please people, she will try and keep up a youthful veneer, (rather than holistic health) for as long as possible.

The Keeper's Hurdles

The Keeper's core desire is to steward the gift of the one body she has been given. She is vigilant and alert, bent on doing what she should because it is right. The Keeper experiences the most stress when she feels unhealthy. She can release the temporary happy neurochemicals of serotonin, which imbue a positive outlook on life, by pursuing a meaningful challenge. Creating and focusing on a long-term fitness Joy Goal as her challenge is crucial to her success. Let's take an inventory of the Keeper's common hurdles along the path and ways of clearing each one for joy!

Hurdle #1

Exercise is purely duty-driven.

Hurdle for joy: *Focus on the long-term fulfillment.* One of my friends' favorite physical activities was biking, but he has since fallen out of any sort of exercise habit. Recently he started working out at the gym, and I asked him why—what was his newfound motivation? I listed a few potential reasons, but he couldn't identify with any of them. "I don't really find any happiness in fitness. It doesn't make me confident, energetic, balanced, or capable of managing stress—it is a matter of doing something that will hopefully make me less incompetent as I age. It isn't something I *want* to do, but something I feel like I should/need to do. As another friend said, 'I work out so I don't end up 65 and unable to stand up from the toilet.'"

I laughed at his honesty and responded, "It sounds like you workout because it's the right thing to do, even if you don't like it. Regardless of motivation, you'll have more strength because you're exercising to enjoy your life and the people in it. And maybe you view exercise like I do with cleaning—I don't *like* to clean, but do it because it helps my family and the people who come to our house. Is that basically how you feel about exercise?"

He confirmed: "Cleaning is the perfect analogy."

Even though I don't enjoy cleaning while I do it, I've found joy in it by turning on my favorite dance music. I always experience the reward of achievement for the good of others when I see the finished result. Focusing on the longer-term Joy Goal is a useful step in practicing delayed gratification and strengthens your willpower in the moment. Even if you are unable to find one thing to enjoy about exercise *while* you do it (refer to the Bonus Chapter at the end of this book on ways to spark joy), know that Jesus is with you regardless and it's still bonding time with Him.

What is one thing you can enjoy about exercise?

_____

_____

_____

What is one long-term benefit?

_____

_____

_____

Who will it positively affect besides yourself?

_____

_____

_____

Hurdle #2

You avoid exercise for fear of reinjury.

Hurdle for Joy: *Take small steps.* Biomechanist Katy Bowman sets up a scenario in her book *Whole Body Barefoot* of how we position our bodies when we think we are going to get hurt, and likens it to the posture of an elderly person who has had experience with falling and has greater fear of falls because of brittle bones. Imagine yourself walking on an icy sidewalk. How do you change your posture and gait? Typically, we bend our knees to lower our centers of gravity in case of a fall, shift our feet along stiffly to create less flexion in our ankles, and tense our shoulders to brace our arms to catch ourselves, just in case. But once you get injured, more surfaces and movements can start to look icy. Craig Williamson explains the memory-pain connection in his book *Muscular Retraining for Pain-Free Living:*

> *If you experience pain every time you raise your left arm above your shoulder, you naturally expect to feel the same pain when you raise your arm again. Underneath this expectation is your memory of pain. This memory causes your muscles to contract, which then can cause the same pain every time you raise your arm over your shoulder. So your anticipation of pain makes it more likely that you will end up having pain. Frequently, people mistake this situation for one in which there is an actual structural problem or injury.[83]*

His solution is to preach truth to yourself whenever you start to feel the pain where there is no injury. Tell yourself that it is *not* injured, and then list the medical reasons why you are healthy. The mental reinforcement aids in the physical healing.

If you are injured, please consult with a health professional. If cleared of injury, begin building your faith little by little with small movements just outside your comfort zone but within a safe range of motion. This will help to break those bonds of immobility with associated memories of injury. You will slowly regain your strength, partly by circulating blood flow to the area, until you are strong enough in mind and body.

If anxiety over reinjury is blocking your way, turn it into excitement. The physical response to anxiety and excitement as a result of adrenaline—faster breathing, flushed face, sweaty palms—are the same, but what's different is mindset. An anxious mindset says, "I'm going to get hurt again," while an excited mindset of hope thinks, "This could be the day I feel better!" Set the joy of hope before you, pushing fear aside and keeping Jesus in the forefront of your mind.

One more way to strengthen yourself mentally is not just looking ahead, but looking around at role models of health. There are plenty of people who aren't afraid to use their bodies well into old age. Take Jean Calment, for example. Calment was a French woman who lived to be 122 years of age. She took up fencing at age 85 and continued to ride her bicycle up until her 100th birthday![84] If she can do it, why can't we?

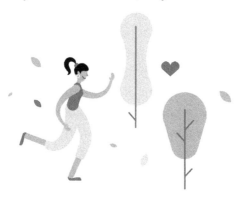

What's one thing you've been wanting to try but fear of injury has stopped you? Are you physically strong enough to try a small dose?

_____

_____

_____

_____

_____

Hurdle #3:

> *"All or nothing" syndrome. If all the stars aren't aligned, if the right outfit isn't clean, or the workout needs to be cut shorter than usual, you might think it's not worth doing it at all.*

Hurdle for Joy: *Every step counts.* A marathon is not won by speed, but perseverance. The competitor is not disqualified for stopping for a break, or even restarting. The only requirement is that while she runs, she stays on the course. In your fitness journey, know that every little bit and bout of movement you do adds up. Even a short period of exercise is extremely beneficial.

Studies have shown that if someone has been sedentary, the first twenty minutes of movement provides most of the health benefits, including prolonged life and reduced disease risk.[85] Don't overthink it—set a twenty minute timer and get moving before you change your mind! While twenty minutes of sustained activity provides the most benefits for the heart, making movement a lifelong rhythm means making it as normal as brushing your teeth. Instead of planning the perfectly tailored workout as a detour for your day, make the habit to move a more natural part of your habitat. The book *Blue Zones* outlines the nine lifestyle habits shared by people around the world who live the longest, and one of the habits is to Move Naturally.

"The world's longest-lived people don't pump iron, run marathons or join gyms. Instead, they live in environments that constantly nudge them into moving without thinking about it. They grow gardens and don't have mechanical conveniences for house and yard work."[86]

You don't need to spend any extra money or even go out of your way to make movement a normal part of your day. You could switch out your driving commute for a more mobile route and reap the benefits of being outside and improving your health. People who walk to work were also 17 percent less likely than people who drive to have high blood pressure. Cyclists were around half as likely to have diabetes as drivers.[87] If your work is too far away, drive part of the way and walk the rest. Walking is a great opportunity to be with the Lord before diving into work, lifting up prayers of thanksgiving and petitioning to prepare you for the next assignment.

Hurdle #4

> *Taking health scores personally. If a BMI*
> *measurement says you're obese, or heart rate*
> *test says your scores are below average, it*
> *may feel like an attack on your identity.*

Hurdle for Joy: *Take a higher perspective.* This is a good time to ask the question, "But how do I feel emotionally and mentally?" Biohealth markers are only one external part of our holistic selves. With the same vigor you use to take care of your physical health, begin to monitor the other integral components of your health.

On a scale of 1-5, 1 being poor and 5 being excellent, how would you rate your:

Physical health

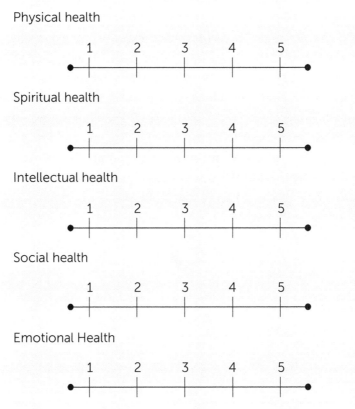

Spiritual health

Intellectual health

Social health

Emotional Health

If you scored a 2 or lower on any of the above categories, write one healthy next step you can take next to it.

No matter what how you score above, God will not score us on our health on Judgment Day. He will take into account how well we stewarded what we were given according to His scales, which are justice and mercy. We are justified in Christ and given what we need in Him. So let's take hold of His health for us now!

Hurdle #5

> **Relying on your own efforts. You do a lot to stay**
> **healthy for the long haul. But do you ever feel dismayed**
> **when you run out of your own strength or frustrated**
> **when people get in the way of your health pursuit?**

Hurdle for Joy: *Pick Three.* Instead of trying to be 100% healthy 100% of the time, the fitness motivation book *No Sweat* suggests focusing on your top three health priorities in order (e.g. sleep, physical movement, time alone). These are the three things that if you don't do, you don't feel like yourself. For a fun exercise, ask your loved ones about their top three, write them down at the same time, then flip over your papers and compare answers. You might be surprised at the differences! Find ways to help each other incorporate them and guard your everyday priorities.

What are your top three health priorities for your day?

_____

_____

_____

_____

_____

This is certainly not an exhaustive list of common barriers for the Keeper. He will be tempted to overthink every obstacle in front of him, circling it to see every angle, performing a risk analysis before attempting a jump. The word "hurdle" as both a description of the obstacle and a solution will help explain how the Keeper can ultimately master his hurdles. When (not if) he trips over a hurdle, the Keeper can be comforted by knowing that stumbling is for sanctification: "And some of the wise shall stumble, so that they may be refined, purified, made white, until the time of the end, for it still awaits the appointed time" (Daniel 11:35). He can get a running start for each hurdle with faith knowing that whether he clears it or not, he has succeeded. And that brings him joy!

Invest in the Greater Home

We may be able to clear small hurdles, make progress, and make renovations and additions on the home of our body, like plastic surgery or knee replacements. But at the end of our time on Earth, we will lose this body to gain a glorified one. Alisa Keeton, the founder of Revelation Wellness, has recently faced this hard truth head-on and has chosen to invest in her eternal home while she honors this temporary one, for as long as the Lord gives it to her, as an offering to Him:

> I have to continually fight the lie (especially as I get older) that I am 'losing it' and 'not who I once was.' And the truth is... I AM! If 'it' is defined as physical ability and the boundless energy of my youth, than yes... I am losing 'it.' And that has to be okay.
>
> I am thankful for the ability to see my body as my vessel for a glorious vision and not just a vehicle to pay the bills or win approval. Let's just say, like a good financial planner, I have learned to diversify my investments. My time and energy are best spent on eternal things. I cash in daily on unsinkable hope, radical grace, and a future that no demon in hell or muscle lost on earth can keep me from.
>
> A little less muscle tone in exchange for a bigger vision and healing love for others who hurt? Worth it!

Now, I move my body six days a week..maybe. Give or take depending on the day, week, or season. And I don't do it because I have to. I do it because God loves to talk with me when I move, whether I am in or out of yoga pants.

I'm officially the CEO of my life: body, soul and Spirit. I'm a woman whom the Lord has brought a long way from lying half dead on a couch, ripped and lean, to a fully alive woman who is able and ready to rise to love.[88]

Eventually, we all fall short of every worldly standard for health. But just as my pregnant body was a home for my baby, the Lord is our home. The Keeper needs to connect her fitness motivation to the praise of her Creator to complete her joy.

Complete Your Joy: Live for the Creator's Praise

In the parable of the talents, each of the three men are given different treasures, as we are each given unique bodies with varying abilities and capacities. The master of the house praises those who invested their talents by saying, "Well done, good and faithful servant. You have been faithful over a little; I will set you over much. Enter into the joy of your master." (Matthew 25:21). But the servant who buried his talent did not trust the Master, but thought him to be a "hard man." Instead of seeing the Master as generous, he viewed him as demanding and did nothing with the talent, leaving it to rust in the ground, until the master called him to account.

Jesus, on the other hand, knew that harsh thoughts about God come from a hard heart. Jesus was deeply aware of the loving nature of His Father, who publicly proclaimed His love:

"You are my Son, whom I love; with you I am well pleased."
LUKE 3:22

"This is my Son, whom I have chosen; listen to him."
Luke 9:35

Jesus, the Beloved, volunteers to become human, takes the curse of sin and death on the cross, and is broken for our acceptance. Jesus is *your* living affirmation that the Father loves you.

"...but God shows his love for us in that while we were still sinners, Christ died for us."
Romans 5:8

We don't have to strive to keep up, to be affirmed, or to be valued according to how healthy we are. God accepts you *as you are.* He thinks you're a Keeper! His unbreakable love allows you to live out of His praise, and empowers you to move for joy, because you're worth investing in. Since Jesus was broken, we don't have to fear the breakdown of our body. It is only when a muscle tears that it grows back stronger. It is only when we are broken that we will multiply. It is only when we lose our lives that we will save them.

The Keeper's key to sustaining heavenward health is to listen to the Lord. First, hear Him when He says He loves you. Then you can trust Him as the shepherd of your health. By walking in step with His Spirit, you will not only reach your Joy Goal (according to His guidance), but have the strength in Christ to stand before Him and hear, "Well done, good and faithful servant. Enter into the joy of your master."

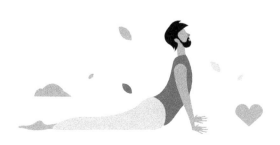

Based on your life thus far, what words do you expect to hear when you give an account for your talents, according to the gospel's perspective?

_____

_____

_____

_____

_____

Practice receiving His unconditional love. Lie flat on the floor. As you inhale, say "Jesus," and on the exhale, say "loves me." He loves you just as you are, without doing a thing. As author Anne Lamott suggests, "We're not what we do, but what we receive."[89]

The Keeper's Core Verse

The Keeper shows reverence for the Lord by respecting her body through a lifetime of exercise. Let's strengthen your core and keep your health together with Scripture training.

> *"So we make it our goal to please him, whether we are at home in the body or away from it."*
> 2 Corinthians 5:9, NIV

The above verse is better read in a slightly larger context within the book of Corinthians, so I've included the surrounding verses here:

> *"Therefore we are always confident and know that as long as we are at home in the body we are away from the Lord. For we live by faith, not by sight. We are confident, I say, and would prefer to be away from the body and at home with the Lord. So we make it our goal to please him, whether we are at home in the body or away from it. For we must all appear before the judgment seat of Christ, so that each of us may receive what is due us for the things done while in the body, whether good or bad." 2 Corinthians 5:6-10, NIV*

Therefore we are always confident and know that as long as we are at home in the body we are away from the Lord. For we live by faith, not by sight: It takes courage to walk by faith, living with the tension that we are not yet with the Lord, but are called to steward the home He has given us. By faith, we know that He knit us together in our mother's womb and will be greeting us after the tomb.

We are confident, I say, and would prefer to be away from the body and at home with the Lord: To be at home in the body means to have a fixed abode, and to be away from the body is to be free from the restrictions of this world and enjoy God's manifest glory. While being "away from the body" is always used positively in the Bible, it does not mean that being in the body is negative. Paul described the tension between yearning for pain-free communion with Jesus and serving in the body like this: "to live is Christ, and to die is gain" (Philippians 1:21). To live as Christ lived is to share the sufferings of the flesh so that we can also share in the joy of His resurrection Spirit. To live as Christ lived is to suffer to serve others and reap joy: "To remain in the flesh is more necessary on your account. Convinced of this, I know that I will remain and continue with you all, for your progress and joy in the faith" (Philippians 1:24-25). The Keeper focuses not on suffering the temporary pain of fitness for her own health, but to be healthy enough to support others.

So we make it our goal to please him: This ambitious phrase "we make it our goal" means to be "zealous, strive eagerly, desire very strongly" or to show affection for what is personally valued.[90] Because Jesus pleased the Father by walking in His will, setting us free from duty-driven obedience and into joy-led movement, God is pleased with us. And so we gain the heart of Jesus to please the Father. This word "to please" is the same word used in Romans 12:1 to offer yourselves as a living sacrifice, holy and acceptable to God. It is also used later in Romans: "For the kingdom of God is not a matter of eating and drinking but of righteousness and peace and *joy* in the Holy Spirit. Whoever thus serves Christ is *acceptable* to God and approved by men." (Romans 14:17-18, emphasis added). Your joyful movement is not only acceptable to Him, but proclaims the Kingdom!

For we must all appear before the judgment seat of Christ, so that each of us may receive what is due us for the things done while in the body, whether good or bad: The Berean Study Bible Translation is this: "that each may *receive back* the things done through the body" (emphasis added). What we reap, we will sow. And God will not judge us based on the facade of our house but the foundation. He will judge us not on the strength of our physical body, but the fortitude of our faith.

Joy Gifts of the Keeper

Knowing your struggles allows you to turn them over to the Lord to become strengths. Receive them, refine them, and share them with others.

- **You are quick to do what is right:** You not only know what is best for your body, but you live it out. Your diligence to wisdom is a well of inspiration for the next generation.

Share this joy gift by telling one other person what you have learned about the eternal benefits of health.

- **You listen to what your body needs:** Abiding by your conscience in how to move is one way of obeying the Lord's voice. The Seventh-day Adventists "believe that the body is the temple of the Holy Spirit, and that God communicates to us through our bodies. So the things you do to impair your thinking and impair your health are cutting you off from God's revelation."[91] You want to walk by faith so you can hear God better.

  Bless with this joy gift by laying hands on someone else in prayer and giving them the Lord's Word.

- **You seek and achieve stability:** By taking care of the one body God has given you, you honor the gift by building a body of strength to withstand years of wear and tear, resilience to disease, and a home for vitality to bring life to others.

  Revitalize another member of the body with this joy gift by bringing life to someone who is in ill health.

A Home with the Lord

When I became pregnant, I became a home for my daughter. Now that she is born, I want to still feel like home for her. A home is a place where you feel loved and accepted, and I want her to know that I love and accept her no matter how she performs. The Lord is our home, and with Him we are always loved and eternally accepted. We exercise out of joyful gratefulness of the gift He has given us in the life that He paid for with His own body. And we can be comforted knowing that even when our earthly body is no longer a fit dwelling for us, we will always have a home with the Lord.

Foundation Exercise

The feet are the foundation of an upright body. Let's practice building our home on the firm foundation Rock of the Lord by fixing our feet.

Position your ankles right underneath your hip bones and point your toes straight forward. Think about your feet as screws, and screw them into the ground externally, feeling the inner arches of your feet lift slightly and your knees engage at your hips, feeling the sides of your glutes activate as well. This provides the most stable position for your body to not only carry its own weight, but to handle the weight of something like a dumbbell, a child, or a heavy bag.

Our feet are the first connection point to the earth. Whenever we stand barefoot and feel the ground beneath us, let this sensation remind us to build our lives on Christ. The sagging effects of gravity no longer have a hold on us when we let the Lord build within us the Kingdom "that cannot be shaken" (Hebrews 12:28) as we stand on the eternal weight of glory.

Keeper Quick Reference Guide

When you need to remember what gets you going, refer to the statements below:

Keeper motivation: Enjoying the Lord through the gift of exercise *is* good stewardship.

Joy declaration: "I will show reverence for the Lord by respecting my body through a lifetime of joy-filled exercise with Him."

Keeper prayers to be used for exercise:
- "All for the Lord."
- "It is finished."
- "Faithful to the end."

If you are a Keeper, you may continue to Chapter Eight to begin conquering your Joy Goal plan.

ACT:
Walk It Out

Chapter Eight

You Were Made For This

Fifty crunches, thirty push-ups, for fifty-five years. I could hear my dad grunting with the effort as he shooed away the dogs that jumped on him during his back-rolling exercises. He did this every morning and every night to protect his back so he could do what brought him joy—having the strength to serve his family, neighborhood, church, and country. Being able to live a pain-free life enabled this Army retiree to coach sports when we were small, take us on neighborhood jogs to pick up trash, make beds for the needy, and rush ahead to open doors for anyone in pubic.

His Joy Goals often stem from the duty-driven Keeper: to steward his body well to be healthy for others. How did this purpose determine his steps? This is what we will explore in the following chapters. This last section of the book will follow the roadmap set forth by Hebrews 12:1-7, looking to Jesus in our call to endure. Chapter Eight will guide you in what to do, Chapter Nine will give you a plan for how to do it, and Chapter Ten will help you adapt it for real life.

To start off, let us determine what to do. Whenever I teach fitness classes, I plan a workout for the people ahead of time, then ask a series of three questions when I arrive. I want you to ask yourself these three questions to set up a workout fit for you.

1. Defense: What do you need to protect?

Question number one: "Are there any injuries I need to be aware of?" We need to first feed the lambs,[92] or tend to the weak members of our body. The enemy will always go for our weak spots first, so we must set up a strong defense to give ourselves time and space to heal. A weak link can break the whole chain.

By treating our weaknesses with kindness, we place trust gates in our fences. When we take steps to protect injuries in a display of how the Lord defends us, we begin to see and trust that we will be taken care of. As a result, we begin to take risks by stepping out of our comfort zones, one confident move at a time. When my dad had back pain, a doctor prescribed him stretching exercises to strengthen and protect his back. Eventually, this defensive measure evolved into a whole calisthenics routine including push-ups and sit-ups. A good defense is the best offense.

When I started developing back pain from abdominal separation after pregnancy, I too was prescribed stretching and strengthening exercises. I had tried dozens of programs, two rounds of pelvic floor and physical therapy, did all the right exercises, and avoided the wrong ones. I used essential oils, increased my gelatin intake to support connective tissue restoration, bought belly bands, girdles, and splints. But with my second pregnancy, it only grew worse. I found myself thinking, "Am I just wasting my time? If it didn't work before, what makes me think it will work now?" I was so ready to be done defending my core and wanted to break out of the gates in a full sprint. My dream of having a strong core shriveled along with my joy. Unbelief lead to inaction, and I slacked off on my physical therapy exercises that week.

Defensive measures can take a lot of time and patience. When returning from an extensive injury, we must fix our eyes on the Lord of living hope instead of standing on our own shaky expectations of what we should be able to do. To be successful in our respective Joy Goals, we must begin with faith in God. Faith lays the foundation of belief to anchor the hope of action for the reward of joy.

> *"Therefore, since we are surrounded*
> *by so great a cloud of witnesses,"*
> HEBREWS 12:1A

It is important to start out knowing that you know you're not going alone. God is the pace car leading the way to your Joy Goal, with a support team of goodness and mercy following after you. He fills the sidelines with faithful cheerleaders, those who have gone before and urge you onwards by their faithful examples. A witness, as referenced in the verse above, is someone who testifies to the truth by his way of life. My dad was one of those for me, and remembering his daily example encouraged me to persevere. Another cheerleader was my physical therapist. She believed that these exercises were my best shot at uniting my core. I believed her, I believed in hope, and the energy of belief to prove them all right was what kept me going. And today, I can't say that my abs are back together. Maybe they won't ever be healed on this side of heaven. But I do feel more put together in body and spirit through the strength of walking in obedience. And maybe that is where true strength rises.

Covering Each Other's Weaknesses

The Warrior knows that we are all members of one body and that all parts are connected. When our faith is weak, we can look to each other for strength. This is why it is important not only to know your own motivator, but how others in your life are uniquely wired. If you haven't already, think about your close friends and family and go read the chapters that you suspect fit them. Feel free to step into their shoes and take the quiz as they would. Then read the descriptions below of what your motivator is prone to believe, and how you can practically support those in your life.

When the Looker believes he doesn't belong, the Warrior links arms with him and invites him to a game of basketball.

When the Freebird believes she will be overcome with stress, the Hero lends a hand and picks up her kids from school so she can have an hour to de-stress at the gym.

When the Hero believes there's no time to take for herself, the Keeper comes up with a self-care schedule tailored just for her, including a daily workout that will fill her up.

When the Warrior can't lift what he used to and believes that nothing is working out for him, the Looker sees his strengths and calls them out, reminding him that his efforts encourage others.

When the Keeper believes she is a failure because she discontinued her set workout plan, the Freebird can remind her that it's right to change course and adapt her plan according to curves in the road of life.

What are your physical weaknesses or limitations?

_____

_____

_____

_____

_____

_____

How are you protecting and supporting them as a reflection of how God loves you?

_____

_____

_____

_____

Whose example of being faithful to staying fit encourages
you, and why?

_____

_____

_____

_____

As a demonstration of how our strengths can cover each
other's weaknesses, put your palms together, fingers
extended to the sky. Notice that in between each set of
fingers, there is a gap. One by one, starting with the index
fingers, pull the matching fingers down to the opposite
hand. When you are done, your hands will be clasped
together. Notice how much stronger this position is, when
each finger covers the opposite gaps. Let it be a reminder
of how we need each other for strength.

2. Discipline: What do you need to do?

The second question I ask my class or clients is: "What do you need to do?" I think we often make joy in fitness more complicated than it needs to be. We think we need to keep up with all the latest trends, we need to meet our activity goals every day, we need to look like the fitness instructor, and we need to be first on the leaderboard. During a healthy living challenge, several women voiced their struggle with the crushing number of options and expectations dumped upon them:

- "I am realizing more and more that I have a problem. I want to lose weight to feel better, have more energy, and be more confident. But I tend to overcomplicate it all. Like with fitness: I obsess that I need a plan to follow, but then find one and can't stick to it because sometimes I just want to go for a walk, so take a detour from the plan. Or, I stumble across other plans and think, 'Maybe that one will hold the key!' Am I putting fitness and weight loss on a pedestal? But wouldn't God want me to lose weight so I can be healthier? Any advice on how to work through all of this?"
- "I am also overwhelmed with all of the different food plans and exercise recommendations... I feel like I have ADD and can't get started and stick with anything."
- "I think we fall off programs because we think if we do it differently for a day we have 'blown it.'"

Have you ever felt like this?

"let us also lay aside every weight,
and sin which clings so closely"
HEBREWS 12:1A

Hebrews tells us that if we want to run the race with endurance, we have to throw off anything extra we don't need. Let's make exercise simple. "Simplicity is freedom. Duplicity is bondage. Simplicity brings joy and balance. Duplicity brings anxiety and fear."[93] Temporary weight adds strength to one's muscles, but if it is not removed, the extra weight debilitates. The author of Hebrews compares our walk of faith with the Spartan-like training of an athlete, like the swimmer who razors away every leg hair just to shave off a millisecond of time on the clock. One commentary explains the metaphor of "every weight" from the verse above further:

> *"The Greek word was sometimes used by Greek writers to denote the excessive size and weight of body which the athlete sought to reduce by means of training; but may also signify the encumbrance of any burden, unnecessary clothing, and the like. It is here best taken in a general sense, as denoting anything that encumbers, and thus renders the athlete less fitted for the race."*[94]

The Christian runner packs light for the long race. She only needs one thing. As the story of Mary and Martha illustrates, her one thing is not a thing at all but an action: to listen to Jesus.

Jesus does things differently. Instead of doing what we've always done, let's clear the board and start fresh, renewing our minds for His plans.

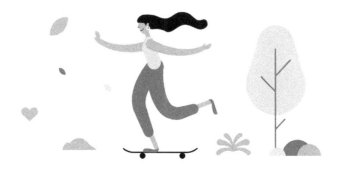

Let's rethink exercises. Is your current routine serving your needs in this season? If not, what will?

_____

_____

_____

_____

Let's rethink exercise clothes. Are you wearing what fits you and the activity at hand? Do you need to upgrade your attire or be more relaxed about it?

_____

_____

_____

_____

Let's rethink your workout space. Dream about your ideal movement center, whether that be a regular indoor facility or a variety of studios and outside environments. How can you make that happen?

_____

_____

_____

_____

Fitness may be different for each bioindividual, but all of us have the same kinesthetic constructs to build from. I like the ACE integrated Fitness Training continuum because it shows how we build on our physical growth from the foundation of function, and it displays our fitness journey as a spectrum instead of a static pyramid. Over time, we get stuck in certain movement patterns that need to be shaken up and settled back down to the body's original design. Before jumping into any new program, let's assess where we are on the continuum and go from there:

1. Function: Focus on stability and mobility training, and building an aerobic base.
2. Health: Add functional and resistance training using body-weight. Work on aerobic efficiency.
3. Fitness: Once your aerobic and resistance base is built, it's safe to gradually add loads to increase your abilities.
4. Performance: Add anaerobic intervals and skills-based training into your program.[95]

Do What You Need First

Think about what you *need* to do to get to your Joy Goal, and do that first. This is an exercise that you don't necessarily enjoy in the moment, but you know it will be immensely beneficial in your life. This includes healing an injury, strengthening a weakness, or simply being more disciplined. I don't always enjoy doing my physical therapy exercises (unless I'm doing them while watching *30 Rock*), but I need to do them to regain function.

One coaching client said, "I used to do group fitness four to five a week because it was fun and it felt good. But now I'm in a time of craving solitude, especially in the summertime. Once you hit forty, your hormones kick in and your body goes soft. I want to get into a regular routine with group fitness or weights to stay strong and try to work in a thirty-minute walk. I know I need discipline."

What do you need for discipline? Let's start out by taking a look at where you spend most of your time and what your body does most of the day. Then we can add in a movement supplement. Since the majority of our time is spent working, read the following occupation categories from the book, *The Pain-Free Program*, and highlight which one fits you:

- *Physical Workers:* Your job requires your body's full attention and may include manual tasks such as lifting, carrying, loading, digging, climbing, bending, crawling, and so forth. Examples include construction, physical therapists, delivery personnel, farmers, and sanitary work.
- *Dexterity Workers:* Your body is still while your hands and fingers do most of the work. Examples of dexterity workers include careers in computers, laboratory workers, dental hygienists, and hairdressers.
- *Multitaskers:* Every day looks different for you, and requires many different body positions. You may be lifting a heavy object one minute and getting into the car the next. Examples include stay-at-home parents, postal workers, restaurant and hospitality workers, and sales jobs.

Knowing your movement needs and current level of daily physical demands informs your exercise program. You may need yoga to help you actively recover from a physically demanding day at work, or if you're a dexterity worker, you'll need to strengthen and mobilize the parts of your body that did not get enough attention.

You might already have an idea of what you need to do to support your Joy Goal, but in case you need some ideas, here are a few activities that line up with each motivator.

Looker:
- *Lift heavy:* anaerobic weight lifting, or heavier resistance training without cardio, improves confidence, rejection resistance, and resilience.
- *Get out:* sunlight produces vitamin D which promotes

serotonin production, the confidence neurochemical. Aim for ten to thirty minutes of midday sunlight every day.
- *Grab a friend:* if classes are intimidating, grab a friend or hire a personal trainer to get into the groove.

Freebird:
- *Ground your live wires:* in the event of a wayward mood, try grounding your joy circuit with the following mindfulness exercises:
  - Overlap your hands together and press them over your heart to feel the beat. Start walking to the beat of your heart and feel how it adapts, reminding you that you can adapt.
  - Walk barefoot in the grass.
  - Awaken your whole body by extending and flexing each joint, starting with your feet all the way up to your head.
- *Interior retreat:* Choose any form of retreat whether that's into your mind like yoga, breathing meditation, or losing yourself to the rhythm of dancing.
- *External retreat*: Get outside of your environment like going for a walk, run, hike, bike, or other outdoor activity.

Hero:
- *Variety of movement:* For a creativity boost, add in linear, multiplanar, and cross-directional exercises to bridge both sides of the brain and integrate imaginative thought with executive strategy. For an example of each, try performing a forward lunge (linear), side lunge (multiplanar), and curtsy lunge (cross-directional). Do movements like these within three hours of a creative endeavor for the most effective results.
- *Move for more brain cells*: Exercise, in all forms, can stimulate something called BDNF in our brains. It stands for Brain Derived Neurotrophic Factor. This protein

promotes the survival of nerve cells (neurons) by playing a role in the growth, maturation (differentiation), and
maintenance of these cells. Exercise at sixty to seventy
percent of your heart rate for twenty to thirty minutes
before a big meeting or learning course to expand your
capacity to take in and apply new information.

- *Submaximal output:* Moderate levels of walking, interval training, Pilates, spinning, and bodyweight strength
exercises are bound to increase energy without leaving
you feeling depleted afterwards.

Warrior:

- *Set and achieve a goal:* The warrior seeks the accomplished
effects of dopamine. Go into every workout with a specific
goal to reach, whether that be a time to beat, a mindfulness activity to focus on, or a certain number of exercises
to complete. Consider joining a thirty-day challenge or
trying a gym with built-in competition, like heart rate
monitoring or posting performance on a board.
- *Exercise with someone:* Make a point to work out in the
physical presence others, whether that is joining a running
club, simply going to a gym where others are working
out, or at home with a neighbor to release oxytocin and
experience human connection to get connected with the
body of Christ.
- *Get out of your comfort zone:* To get a surge of adrenaline,
do something a little out of the ordinary for you, like hiking
a new location, trying a different fitness studio, joining a
sports team, or signing up for a skill-specific series like
boxing or karate.
- *Join the kids:* If you're a parent whose kid is involved in a
sport that offers classes or teams for adults, get in on the
fun and try it out. They might even offer a family discount!

Keeper:

- *Moderate-intensity aerobic exercise:* One-hundred fifty minutes per week (about thirty minutes five days a week) of aerobic exercise may slow down the aging of cells[96] in addition to benefiting the cardiovascular system. Include cycling, swimming, or speed walking into your day at a pace which makes it harder to hold a conversation, or fifty to seventy percent of your maximum heart rate (approximately 220 minus your age).

- *Change your environment:* Make your surroundings suitable for natural movement. Put the most used items in harder-to-reach places, and reduce the use of technology.

- *Be all-inclusive:* In addition to aerobic exercise, add resistance training for bone strength. These can be simple bodyweight exercises like squats, push-ups, and planks. You may do these with little to no break in between, which would count as anaerobic training and improves stamina and speeds fat loss.

Once you decide what you need to do, I recommend doing that first thing in the morning or first in your workout. For example, if you know you need to get your legs strong for an upcoming hike, but hate resistance training, do weighted step-ups first, followed by an activity you like to do, such as running. That activity can be your reward, or the joy set before you, to get you through the part you consider to be discipline. This is also where you will need that faithful cloud of witnesses you can look to for inspiration and lean on for support.

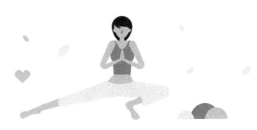

What do you need to do to get you to your Joy Goal?

_____

_____

_____

_____

_____

_____

3. Design: What do you want to do?

The third question I ask my classes or clients after injuries and needs is, "What do you want to do?" Most people kind of shrug, because this answer isn't as obvious. C.S. Lewis explains why joy sounds so muffled: "We can ignore even pleasure. But pain insists upon being attended to. God whispers to us in our pleasures, speaks in our conscience, but shouts in our pains: it is his megaphone to rouse a deaf world."[97] Adults become less sensitive to the voice of joy, especially in exercise, because we become so accustomed to listening to the needs of others and taking care of everyone else. But just imagine that Jesus is looking you in the eyes and asking you, "What do you want me to do for you?" He wants you to be joyful in exercise, because joy in hardship is communion with Christ, and a simple act of smiling through squats can be a beacon of God's Kingdom in a suffering world.

During one coaching call I asked the question, "What do you *want* to do for exercise?" After giving it some thought, the woman on the other line said, "Hm...I don't know. Well, I used to love going on hikes. But now, it feels like a luxury that's out-of-reach. Taking time to do what I want to do feels selfish. It also wasn't modeled well for me, but I know I need to model this well for my kids." We may feel like joy doesn't have a place in the no-nonsense life of adulthood, but to quote C.S. Lewis again: "Joy is the serious business of heaven."

For the Looker: Nourish your inner worth. Do not skip out on something fun that you think others would point and laugh at. Get in the front of that Jazzercise class and own those dance moves! Instead of looking to the mirror, peers, family, friends, or culture for visual approval, remember who you are and whose you are. You are holy, beloved, and chosen in Christ. He sees you, and that frees you to radiate the strength of someone who stands firm in her identity.

For the Freebird: Don't mistake responsibility for a prison, and sulk inside because you are an adult and need to clean the house. Use your Freebird creativity to make cleaning into an exercise game. You don't need to escape your life to feel freedom. You are a temple of the Holy Spirit, who makes you whole right where you are and gives you everything you need when you ask. Make it a point to regularly meet with God in the space of your body and find the freedom of peace so you can help others find that same joy of contentment.

For the Hero: Don't try to fix everyone and everything before you do something fun. Leave the house a mess and take the crying kids outside for a water balloon fight. Leave the email pile and go explore a new area of the office. Don't work harder, work smarter. Know what's yours to own for the day, and only do the activity you need to to support those priorities. If you want to do more, great! Let it be done in joy.

For the Warrior: Use your imagination to turn ordinary movements into extraordinary feats. Imagine your mountain climbers are helping you get up Mount Everest, visualize competing against Tour de France cyclists while on a spin bike, take down the fictional boxing opponent in the ring while throwing punches on a bag. The Warrior also loves company, but don't be discouraged from fitness if you can't get a whole soccer team together to play. Just find one other person. You, one other, and the Lord is an army!

For the Keeper: It's okay if you don't have a perfect plan—just get your tennis shoes on, go outside, and figure out what feels good to you. By remembering that Christ is your righteousness, you're doing it right. If you can't remember what's fun, think about what you liked to do as a kid or what you would do if you had a free day. Enjoying exercise is not just frivolous fun, but reduces stress and prolongs your life.

Maybe you doubt that there's any form of fitness that makes you happy. Maybe you feel like you've tried everything and written off athletics entirely. But perhaps digging into your original design can help, so let's take a deeper look into our ancestry. I'm not talking about a general "let's do what the ancestors did" approach, but a more specific look at your own lineage. Our society is more global, transient, and mobile today, but I believe each of our bodies has adapted to a specific set of motor skills that helped us survive in the past and can bring us joy where we are now. To back up this theory, I'll cite a study from book *Grace, Food, and Everything in Between*[98] about how we are literally healthier when we take enjoyment in family traditions:

> *One study looked at two groups of women from two different cultures. They fed each group a traditional meal and looked at the rate of their iron absorption. Then they fed each group the other culture's traditional food, something*

they weren't as inclined to enjoy, and looked at the rate of iron absorption again. As anticipated, the women absorbed the most iron from their culture's traditional meal. This is to be expected. Our body gets used to the foods we feed it and can better digest something eaten regularly because it has the right enzymes and bacteria to do the job. The interesting part of this study is what happened next. The researchers provided each group of women their own traditional meal, but blended it up in a smoothie. We would think that breaking down the food before feeding it to the women would enhance absorption, making the nutrients in the food more readily available to the body, however the fact that the food was now an unappealing pile of mush ensured that the women were not enjoying their meal as much. The result? They did not absorb near as much iron as they did when they enjoyed what they ate. This may partly explain why different cultures can enjoy completely different diets and still be extremely healthy.

We can apply what we have learned from this study to our movement patterns as well. Just as the women benefited more from traditional food they enjoyed, perhaps we can benefit more from traditional movement we enjoy. One obvious way we benefit is to want to move more, and to move more of our parts, making our physiology more well-rounded, stable, and fit for action. Let's take a brief look at how you were designed and find some ways you were made to enjoy movement.

Heritability and Height

You could take an ancestry.com test, but chances are you can figure out your traits by taking a look at your family tree. The National Institutes of Health reports on the heritability (or likelihood of genetic characteristic being passed on to the next generation) of athletic abilities:

- The heritability of athletic status is around 66%
- The chance that a tall stature will be passed on is about 80%
- The somatotype, which includes bone structure, body composition, metabolic and muscle adaptations, is highly heritable

Our body morphology, or bone structure, determines our height, shoulder width, hip width, limb length, and hand and feet breadth, all of which contribute to athletic abilities. To keep this list short, we will only list the general characteristics and suitable sports for each height range.

Shorter than 5'4"
- Greater strength-to-weight ratio gives you an advantage in weight-lifting competitions divided by weight class
- Greater power-to-weight ratio is helpful for pushing heavy strollers up hills or sprinting short distances
- Faster rotational capability for showing off your triple axle on the ice skating rink, twists from the high dive, flips across the gymnastics floor, or BMX tricks off the ramp
- Greater agility to master tire runs in boot camp class, duck from opponents on the soccer field, or jump out of the way in dodgeball
- Greater balance and lower center of gravity for holding advanced yoga poses or standing your ground in a wrestling match

Taller than 5'4"
- Greater absolute strength for loading up the bar with plates
- Greater work capacity for partner sled pulls
- Greater power for rowing, pole vaulting, or hitting with more torque and sharp angles such as in volleyball
- Greater endurance for the Saturday running club

- Longer arms for basketball and/or legs for hurdles
- Longer forearms to increase the force of the whipping motion when throwing
- Larger hands for catching incoming sports balls
- Bigger feet for pressing off ground while running or as flippers for swimming

Which sports are you better at?

_____

_____

_____

_____

_____

Are there any you would like to try based on your height advantages?

_____

_____

_____

_____

_____

Genetic Heritage

Our bodies are adept at certain sports for play, and it's also likely that we have adapted those traits from certain environments for survival. Because as we know from Chapter Two, joy is inherent to the survival of a species. It's not only beneficial to be able to run fast after our food, but the joy running produces makes us want to do it more and provide for the greater society. And the two go together, since we usually enjoy what we are good at. Your generational origins may explain certain physical giftings, why you have them, and most likely why you enjoy that particular movement.

Natives in the Arctic region have short, stocky bodies, ideal for insulating oneself against the brutal cold and keeping the limbs close to the core, the body's central heating system. Populations who live closer to the equator are taller, which helps distribute heat over a larger surface area to cool the body more quickly. Longer limbs also help reach fruit in tall trees that grow in warm climates. If you are shorter, with a lower center of gravity, you might have ancestry from a colder climate to be better at balancing on surfaces like ice. According to the book *Sports Gene*, body mass and fat mass is inversely related to the mean annual temperature of where that person (or their ancestors) lives.

If you want to take a deeper dive, feel free to take a genetics test, or research "body morphology and athletic ability." Your search will result in fun quizzes like, "Which Olympic sport fits your body?"[99] and scholarly articles titled, "Body physique and dominant somatotype in elite and low-profile athletes with different specializations" that detail body types of endomorphs, ectomorphs, and mesomorphs.[100] But a word of warning if you follow that rabbit trail. You don't want to pin yourself into a box and think that you are only made for certain sports based on physical characteristics. The Freebird might remind you that joy is not rigid, but flexible according to your mood and season. Don't be afraid to try something completely new!

Do you have any insight into your ancestry? Does it help explain the way you were made and what you're good at?

_____

_____

_____

_____

_____

John Calvin said, "Nearly all wisdom we possess, that is to say, true and sound wisdom, consists of two parts: the knowledge of God and of ourselves."[101] I hope that through this chapter, you have learned more about God and yourself: the importance of acting in faith, discerning where you need discipline, and what brings you joy in fitness. Do what you need, what you want, and do more of it. Be more physically engaged with your life and what you love. Your joy and God's glory depends on it!

Exercise

My dad did the same exercises for over fifty years through thick and thin. Depending on his season, he swapped various movements fit for his design and then added the appropriate amount of discipline when needed, like modifying for injuries and sickness. Let's surround ourselves with a great cloud of witnesses (or call to mind the ones we already have) and develop a simple practice of our own. It doesn't have to be the same thing every day, but a regular routine does help to take the thinking out of the equation. Look around to see who inspires you, why, and add in your own body's wisdom about what you need.

What can you do today to begin? The simplest exercise is to take a walk. You may pick a consistent time of day, or set a timer for how long you'll be out there, if that helps to guard yourself from overthinking it. Any athletic effort stems from the lower brain, the "just do it" mental-ity that can be hindered by the higher reasoning of risks and doubts of the upper brain. Don't even call it a work out. Just go and move with thanksgiving, focusing less on performance and more on creativity and experimentation, exploring how God designed you. The more you do, the easier it will be to find your groove and your joy.

Chapter Nine

Create Your Joy Goal Plan

"How are you doing?" I asked the girl as I caught up with her at a 5K race. "Just trying to get through this," she answered through gritted teeth, not even glancing at me. I can take a hint. She wanted to be left alone, so I ran ahead, passing a younger boy who had started walking. When he heard my footsteps behind him, he shot a paranoid glance over his shoulder, charged into a sprint for about ten yards, and slowed back down to a walk, looking down in disappointment. I noticed him doing this with each person who passed him. These two runners symbolize two approaches to endurance: grin and bear it because life is hard, or let others set the pace for your race because the finish line is too far. I've realized that adults have trained for endurance, but lack joy. Kids have joy, but little endurance. We need both! We need to be able to make it for the long haul, and to experience joy on the way.

In the previous chapter, you discovered what you need and want to do, and now you will create a flexible plan for your Joy Goal that will endure throughout your season.

Training Endurance and Cultivating Joy

"let us run with endurance..."
HEBREWS 12:1A

There are very few things we are willing to do for an extended period of time, especially if they are uncomfortable like running.

But even running can be joyful when we train for it. Every time our minds tell us to stop and we keep going, we overcome a mental obstacle and our faith grows stronger. Training for endurance in a disposable, replaceable, quick-to-become-obsolete society isn't easy. Investing in a body that will last a lifetime while refining a soul that will last an eternity is incredibly countercultural. Endurance training lays the groundwork for durable joy!

Endurance is literally easier for some people. Physical endurance is fueled by slow-twitch muscle fibers, the kind that are recruited during aerobic exercise and burn carbohydrates and lipids to generate oxygen in the cells. We are each born with a different amount of fast-twitch (those that engage during quick power movements like sprinting) and slow-twitch fibers, but studies show that women have more of these fibers than men and display more of a "fatigue resistance."[102] Could it be that women are designed with more endurance fibers to sustain the marathon of labor? And that men have more fast-twitch fibers to sprint to the shop and get the woman a giant smoothie aftwards? This is a personal theory, but a highly tenable one, am I right? While we cannot add more type I endurance muscle fibers to our original design, we *can* convert type IIb fast-twitch fibers into moderate fast-twitch type IIa fibers (more suited for endurance) by working on extending our aerobic capacity in longer bouts of submaximal effort and through resistance training.[103]

This shows we can enhance our physical endurance, and every step counts: "Taking chances, even small, mundane ones, is how we learn to navigate the world. Each time you try something new, your brain releases dopamine, the pleasure-and learning-hormone."[104] If dopamine is experiencing pleasure through learning, then even as adults we can experience the joy of a child by greeting each training session as a teacher of endurance. Read what God has been showing Stephanie through a new practice of jogging:

I've never been a jogger. I enjoy cardio kickboxing and biking. Yet, here I am, jogging and doing it with joy. I smile as I do it, too. I'm realizing that nothing I dream of or hope for is random. I've always dreamed of jogging and having that type of endurance. Slowly, without realizing, I see God winking at me as if He is reminding me He hears me and knows my deepest longings. If He can help me in these smaller things, I know He's even more willing to help me in the bigger things.

Nothing is impossible! As the Lord is gradually growing Stephanie's trust in Him through every step she takes on her runs, I pray that God will use every step of your physical training with Him to expand your faith and increase your joy.

Do you need more endurance training or joy in the moment? How would this specialized training better equip you for this season?

_____

_____

_____

_____

_____

Your Seasonal Joy Goal Plan

"...the race that is set before us..."
HEBREWS 12:1

The Greek word used here for *race* means "a gathering, a contest, a struggle." Whenever we start to feel stuck in our struggle, it may be because the path has turned and the old ways are no longer working. The secret to enduring success is not just in forming habits over a period of twenty-one days, but forming habits specific to your season of life. When researching how long it takes for someone to form a habit, every scrap of research cited different numbers, but one piece of truth stood out among the rest: "while individual times could vary."[105] And the good news about forming a new *exercise* habit is physical movement restructures the brain over time, as it "triggers new cell growth in the memory, motor function, and executive functioning parts of the brain."[106]

While I love planning my days, weeks, and months, I have started to realize the value in planning for life seasons instead of following the calendar year. For instance, New Year's goals aren't always effective because our seasons of life do not always coincide with January first. My nine-month season of pregnancy put all kinds of new demands on my body, and none of them lined up with my previous calendar plans. If we want to run with endurance for the race marked out for us, we will reverse engineer our current season of life. I have outlined a guide below to help you create your seasonal plan based on your Joy Goal. Let's get started!

1. Recap

What is not working in fitness?

_____

Write down your Joy Goal:

_____

_____

What is your main motivator? Refer to the example chart below, highlight one, then create your own chart.

EXAMPLES

Workouts Not Working	Sample Joy Goal	Motivator
I've tried every workout program before	I want to enjoy my trip to the beach	Confidence of the Looker
I don't enjoy exercising	I need to keep it together during the stress of moving	Peace of the Freebird
Exercise is boring	I want to recover from a rejection	Victory of the Warrior
I don't have time	I need enough energy to take care of kids while I go to school and husband works	Effectiveness of the Hero
I'm too tired	I want to stay strong to play with my grandkids	Stewardship of the Keeper

Workouts not working	Joy goal	Motivator

2. Short Finish Lines

The harder a task is, the more finish lines we need. I won't need
to schedule any picnic breaks into my leisurely walks. But if I am
teaching a High Intensity Interval Training (HIIT) class, breaks
are essential to survive the work. I may divide the class up into
Tabata intervals, which are twenty seconds of a high intensity
exercise, like burpees, followed by ten seconds of rest. Halfway
through the high intensity interval, I'll encourage the class with
the wisdom of the *Unbreakable Kimmy Schmidt*: "You can stand
anything for ten seconds!"[107] Likewise, if you are just starting
out running, you may need to break up your mile-long run into
shorter finish lines. Think about running to the next driveway,
then walking until you get to the next house. Repeat until you
can lengthen your runs to longer finish lines or driveways that
are farther apart.

Sometimes we are exerting ourselves so much that we honestly don't think we can make it until the buzzer or until the
next milestone. When enduring externally is too tough, pull
your efforts inward to focus on your breath, not the timer.
This is a good time to take control of the panic and doubting
by harnessing the proactive power of your rhythmic breath
and connecting it with unceasing prayer. This is the only way
I made it through the half-marathon I trained so poorly for.
When your body says, "I can't!" let this admission be your
prayer of petition, and allow God's power to become perfect
in your weakness.

Take a moment to apply this by deepening your diaphrag-
matic breathing. Lift the corners of your mouth and inhale
through your nostrils, expanding the breath all the way around
your ribs from the front to the back. Let this inhale expand your
faith and push out the fear that you can't, but He can. And as you
exhale, as though you are blowing through a straw, be reminded
that the way that leads to life is hard and narrow.

Here are each motivator's favorite ways to stay in the zone during a tough workout:

- **The Looker** does best when she can *see someone* doing the exercise with her.
- **The Freebird** is carried through the workout with *rhythm*, whether that's moving through inhales and exhales, or the beat of the music.
- **The Hero** needs a *timer* to keep her on track.
- **The Warrior** keeps going with a *competitor* by his side.
- **The Keeper** likes having continual guidance from a *coach*.

Plan Your Ideal Week

Thinking about staying fit for life feels overwhelming, but when we break up our lives into decades, years, months, and weeks, we can better focus on what we need. Making yourself work out every day can be discouraging because we don't often hit all our body parts in one day, and we need to leave time to rest. Planning your fitness goals over a week's time is more realistic. Think about your seasonal Joy Goal finish line as you walk through the following steps.

Include Discipline, Design, and Rest

1. *What you need to do:* Include what you *need* to do to support your Joy Goal in regular doses. This is your endurance training. For example: If my Joy Goal is to ride a motorcycle cross country, I need to train my upper body two to three times a week (true client story).
2. *What you want to do:* Plan at least one physical activity per week you *want* to do and can look forward to, and keep the child-like joy going. Review Chapter Eight for more ideas on design and discipline.
3. *Rest:* There needs to be at least one day built into the schedule where no workout is required. Rest is essential

for muscle growth! You are still welcome to do any movement of choice, but as the Sabbath is a day of rest, may
it be a day of no obligations. If you want to do a workout, make it light, easy, altogether enjoyable, and full
of praise.

How Much Exercise You Need

Whenever I plan a workout program (or supplemental exercise)
for someone, I go by the FITT principle: Frequency, Intensity,
Time, and Type. According to the 2008 Physical Activity Guidelines, "most health benefits occur with at least 150 minutes
(two hours and thirty minutes) a week of moderate intensity
physical activity, such as brisk walking. Additional benefits
occur with more physical activity." But don't go crazy. Benefits
start to decline after ninety consecutive minutes of activity.
Variety and moderation are our friends! As for type of exercise, the guidelines continue: "Both aerobic (endurance) and
muscle-strengthening (resistance) physical activity are beneficial."[108] And just to be clear, that's two-and-a-half hours of
moderate aerobic exercise, or seventy-five minutes of intense
exercise performed in a minimum of ten-minute sessions, *plus*
two weekly sessions of weight training involving all muscle
groups. To make resistance exercises easy to remember, think
of including movements that utilize hip hinging like a squat,
pushing like in a push-up, pulling as in rowing, and carrying
heavy things to engage your core in each session (hinge, push,
pull, carry).

Progress Your Workouts

The three principles of motivation according to the book *Drive*[109]
are purpose, autonomy, and mastery. Your purpose is your Joy
Goal, autonomy is feeling confident enough to do it on your

own (you may need to ask for help here at first), and mastery is progressing the program. As author Daniel Pink says, "Getting better at something provides a great source of renewable energy." As you set and master progressive goals, that's exactly what you're creating.

Start slow and easy, something even below your perceived ability, at least for the first week. Gradually add in difficulty until you find your flow. You must have the following three factors to achieve flow:

1. A clear goal: this is your Joy Goal.
2. Immediate feedback: noticing cause-and-effect with movements, such as clenching a fist to land a harder hit, or pushing off the ground more to jump higher.
3. Ability meets the demands: too high of a demand results in anxiety, while too high of an ability leads to boredom. Continue adding intensity until you find your limit and reach a balance between the two. If you haven't reached failure, you haven't reached success. Find the point where you can't do any more (within a pain-free zone), then take one step back.

Work Backwards

If your season has a definitive end date, set a goal at the end and work backwards. Let's say Sally's Joy Goal is to have energy to take care of the kids while her husband works and she takes classes. She is motivated by being effective with her time and relates best with the Hero. To sustain energy throughout the day, she will need to do a quick, high intensity workout in the morning, three times a week, and have a short energy-boosting movement session that includes the kids in the afternoons. She loves boxing class, but her gym doesn't have childcare, and she can only go on the weekend when her husband can watch the kids. Trying to fit in a workout always feels stressful on Tuesdays because that is the day she hosts Bible Study in the morning. This will be her rest day. Here's her sample workout week:

SUN	30 minute family walk
MON	Morning 20 min Interval Training, Afternoon 10 min dance party with kids
TUES	Rest Day
WED	Morning 20 min Interval Training, Afternoon 10 min dance party with kids
THU	30 min morning stroller walk up hills
FRI	Morning 20 min Interval Training, Afternoon 10 min dance party with kids
SAT	Boxing class at the gym

If she had no regular activity in her life, she would be starting from the "Function" step in the ACE health continuum. The 15-week semester marks the end of her season, so she would divide up the weeks and reverse engineer her plan:

1. Week 15: Move for 30 minutes a day, 6 days a week
2. Week 12: Move for 30 minutes a day, 5 days a week
3. Week 9: Move for 25 minutes a day, 4 days a week
4. Week 6: Move for 20 minutes a day, 4 days a week
5. Week 3: Move for 15 minutes a day, 3 days a week
6. Week 1: Move for 10 minutes a day, 3 days a week

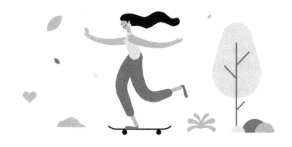

Starting backwards from the end of your season, write down an incremental plan for yourself, as modeled above:

_____

_____

_____

_____

_____

_____

Fill in your workout plan you can start on next week. The first one is your Survival Week—the amount of exercise you need to survive your day:

SUN	
MON	
TUES	
WED	
THU	
FRI	
SAT	

Now fill in your Ideal Workout Week, the amount of exercise you want to achieve to boost your Joy Goal:

SUN
MON
TUES
WED
THU
FRI
SAT

3. Get Support and Celebrate

To endure in the long run, we need to gather support. To keep the joy alive, we must make it a point to celebrate every milestone!

Set Up Support

If my daughter said, "Can you sign me up for Jiu Jitsu classes?" I would look into the details and see that the program required attendance three times a week for a high price. Before I gave her permission that required a sacrifice on my part, I would ask her to try out a few classes to make sure she liked them. If I saw her face light up during class and talk excitedly about it afterwards, I could conclude that Jiu Jitsu sparked joy for her and was worth investing in. I would say, "Yes! Let's think of a way to make this happen for you." Her joy is mine, too!

Even as adults, we still depend on each other. Taking time

to exercise sometimes means taking time away from someone in your life. If they are skeptical of you taking time to exercise, set up a joy sample. Schedule around any work meetings, secure childcare, and set your alarm. Go on a short trial run. You'll make a joy believer out of them when you return with a spring in your step and kiss on their face (or with more energy to do the dishes). Now you have their full support!

Is there anyone you need to talk to to make this plan happen? It could be a family member, asking for help to watch kids, or it could be you, giving yourself permission to take the time and energy to be intentional with this season of life. Write their names and what you need here:

_____

_____

_____

_____

_____

_____

_____

Get Joy Accountability

Family members may be able to provide support, but they don't always make the best accountability partners. I'm a trainer, but my husband needs a peer who can inspire and influence him in ways I can't. This person for you doesn't even have to like fitness!

One coaching client wanted to listen to spiritual development podcasts during his workouts at home. Since he wasn't working out with anyone, but did have a friend who loved podcasts, I suggested the podcast friend be his accountability partner. The friend wouldn't necessarily ask about his workouts, but he would ask about the podcasts, which the client would only listen to during workouts. Your accountability partner doesn't necessarily have to be someone you work out with, but could be someone who shares an interest that you enjoy only while you work out (like watching a show or listening to music).

Who is one honestly encouraging person that you can share your season, struggle, and plan with? Write her name and what she will hold you accountable for:

_____

_____

_____

_____

_____

Celebrate Joy

Support system, check. Accountability, check.
Next, celebrate!

I asked a few friends how they manage to stick with an exercise program. A few of them credited their successes to the guidance of an outside coach or class. But all of them talked about how when they had a positive experience, they felt more inclined to return. The hardest part was showing up! But after they made it through a challenging kickboxing class, de-stressed in Savasana Pose, or made a new friend, they walked away filled with joy. Their past memory built up future motivation: "Just as joy builds on the past, it borrows from the future. It expects certain things to happen."[110] Don't forget to celebrate every success, to commemorate every little finish line you cross! Marking the good feeling or accomplishment of a workout will establish positive associative memories and keep you coming back for more.

Celebration doesn't have to always happen after the workout. Enter the gates of thanksgiving with a word of praise to set the tone for the whole experience. Here's what each motivator might say as a prayer of thanksgiving in the moment and to celebrate a big Joy Goal milestone:

	Give thanks	Milestone celebration
Looker	"You see me"	Buy yourself new workout clothes
Freebird	"You're with me"	Splurge on a new class
Hero	"You're enough"	Get a massage
Warrior	"Your love doesn't quit"	Go out with friends for smoothies
Keeper	"You approve"	Invest in a course, planner, or fitness app

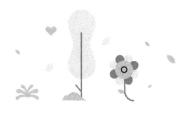

How can you give thanks in the moment and celebrate a big milestone?

_____

_____

_____

_____

4. Modify and Reevaluate

Once you come up with a plan, be free to change it according to your needs. This is where intuitive training comes into play. Just as Jesus meets us where we are, we have the opportunity to meet ourselves where we are at any given time, tune in, and modify our movement plan to release the most joy. This may mean that you need to switch motivator profiles. You can retake the quiz to be sure, and then review that motivator's Quick Reference Guide at the end of the corresponding chapter to set your intentions.

You are also invited to change modes of fitness within your motivator type. What remains constant is your Joy Goal. This means the Looker can quit the gym membership and do at-home workouts because the Lord sees her and has already chosen her whatever she does. She remains focused on His confidence. The Freebird is free to switch out a barre class for a run outdoors, as long as it helps her achieve the peace she seeks. The Warrior can settle for a shorter distance to protect his unstable ankle and still feel victorious in the Lord. The Hero can run in silence instead of multitasking with a podcast, and find just as much joy in learning to be an effective human being for the unseen

Kingdom. The Keeper can veer off from his original workout plan when his health takes a turn and continue to find joy in being a good steward.

Some days might only need slight modifications. A run that worked for you yesterday might feel sluggish today. You might have some extra stress all bunched up in your shoulders. Excess guilt may be keeping you from pursuing joyful movement. Praying something like, "Show me You, show me me," invites the Lord into this process and opens our awareness of Him. Modifying our activity levels as needed is the most effective way to sustain long-term fitness and to stay connected to joy.

Body Scan

If you would like an in-depth assessment, begin with a body scan. Start by lying flat on your back with eyes closed, arms and legs relaxed. Work up from your toes to your head, flexing and releasing, turning and twisting, opening and closing each moveable part. Notice the physical sensations and ponder whether there are any spiritual attachments to each. Are you able to move a joint all around? Praise God for His freedom! What feels unusually tight? Ask the Lord if there are ways you might be shrinking back or held back, and release any striving to let the joy start flowing again. Another method of body scanning is to foam roll. Here you can use outside pressure to test the muscle tightness. If one spot is particularly tense, give it more tender attention by stopping at the trigger point and holding there for thirty to ninety seconds, until the muscle relaxes and pain is reduced.

Once you feel ready, go through the motions of your planned workout. Intuitive training doesn't necessarily mean you don't have any kind of plan. Even Freebirds need structure! Intuitive training is not simply, "do whatever you feel like doing," but "determine what you enjoy, what you need, what your body can handle, and do that." If you have deadlifts on the schedule but found through foam rolling that your hamstrings are particularly tight, consider going lighter than planned and adding in dynamic hamstring stretching throughout the routine.

If you need a more methodical record, an article[111] on intuitive training suggests using the Rate of Perceived Exertion in conjunction with Rate of Technique alongside an exercise program to reinforce constant feedback, reassessment, and redesign of training as it occurs. It's a structured way of staying sober, awake, and alert throughout our movements.

The Rate of Perceived Exertion is placing your efforts on a scale. You could rate it like a review and give it one to five stars, or optimize it from a scale of one to ten (one being, "I'm lying in bed, leave me alone," to ten being "I'm as fast as a cheetah!... but this is not sustainable").

The Rate of Technique is how effectively you are doing an exercise. To do this well, you might need the help of a professional for an initial assessment. At the very least, cut out the distractions and add a mirror or video yourself and play it back to get a more accurate self-assessment. Rate of technique becomes more important when the risk is higher, such as lifting heavier weights, climbing to greater heights, or swimming longer distances.

If you have a written exercise plan, tack these two on to the end of the row where you have written weight / repetitions / sets / time. If you're doing something more informal like a hike, take mental notes on how hard a hill is on your body and if you are moving yourself in an efficient way to master that obstacle. Try writing these observations down until the practice becomes an innate habit.

Reevaluate:
Your season may be indefinite, so set thirty-day milestones to check in with your plan and ask yourself the following questions:

What was successful?

_____

_____

_____

_____

What has changed in your circumstances that you need to adapt to?

_____

_____

_____

If you're not adhering to your plan, is it an obstacle of the heart, a physiological hurdle like modifying a move, or a logistical fix, like figuring out childcare?

_____

_____

_____

_____

Small, Consistent Steps

Sometimes faith calls us to take great leaps, but more often, it requires us to make small, steady steps. Faith calls us to take up our cross daily, to continue following the joy of the Lord, even if He takes us through the valley to get up the mountain. The way we become a regular, joyful exerciser is not by signing up for a gym one time, but through consistent practice. The way we are conformed to the image of Christ is not through a single decision but a lifetime of obedience!

Our bodies form to patterns, not isolated incidents. If we sit in a chair all day, our body's shape will conform to the shape of the chair. We can use the maxim, "You are what you eat," for exercise: "You are how you move." This thinking goes along with the biblical warning to not make idols for ourselves, for, "those who make them become like them; so do all who trust in them" (Psalm 115:8).

We display who or what we trust in by the shape our bodies and souls take. If I have a hard time getting up to move around because my body is stiff from sitting at work, but I fear losing productivity, I show that I am trusting in my work rather than in the Lord to take care of me. If I hesitate to go to an exercise class because I fear others' judgement, that shows I trust in the approval of people rather than God's acceptance of me.

Being consistent doesn't mean doing the same thing every day, but making movement a habit. Eugene Peterson wrote a book called, *Long Obedience in the Same Direction: Discipleship in an Instant Society.*[112] The original book was released in 1980, but think about how much more amplified the word "instant" is in our lives today! When I am able to take a long way, whether that be teaching my daughter how to ride her tricycle on our way to school, or walking to a coffee shop instead of driving, I find that the journey opens my eyes to familiar sights made new, fills my lungs with the fresh air of being present, and refreshes my spirit. By parking farther away, or simply taking more time to walk to a destination, we can make margin in our lives and space to think, pray, plan, and even play! On these routes that take up more time, we might find the endurance and perseverance for the long journey of life. And we might find that the joy is not just at the end, but right there in the middle.

Exercise:

Measure a distance about eight feet long. According to the standards for the standing long jump test[113], covering this distance in one leap is considered excellent. Imagine you're jumping over a creek, to the shore on the other side. Assuming that you have never tried or trained for this test, you have two choices to get across: you can either leap across the eight feet in one jump, or first jump to a log in the creek five feet away. Let's up the stakes: imagine you're also holding $10,000 in your hand. If you do it in one jump, you keep the $10,000. If you jump to the log first, it might tip over and you risk letting go of the money. If you fall in the water, the money could wash away. Which do you choose?

Now test this out on different people in your life: kids, friends, your spouse, maybe even your co-workers. Do their choices reflect their personality? If they took the leap, are they naturally risk-takers or careful and cautious?

Let this be a fun reflection of how we approach the next step on our fitness journeys. If you're more of a risk-taker, consider the cost of your decision and try training for a bigger goal with higher rewards, like training to be able to take the leap in one jump. If you lean toward the calculated end of the spectrum, you're probably one who likes to look at all her options, and noticed the pile of large rocks beside you. You might have taken the rocks and made stepping stones for yourself, ensuring a safe passage, step-by-step. Remember this exercise when you're feeling overwhelmed by decisions. Take stock of your resources, and take the next step toward your Joy Goal.

Chapter Ten

Stay Focused

We were in the home stretch. The finish line was just up ahead, so I urged my then three-year-old daughter to get out of the jogging stroller and finish strong by running beside me. The race wasn't themed, but all life is a stage for her, so she was decked out in her superhero outfit, ready to slay the 5K...except she didn't want to actually run. She wanted to be part of the action, without any action on her part. "But it's too coooollld," she protested under the warmth of the stroller blanket. "When you get out and run, you'll get warm!" I suggested, to which she complained louder. I couldn't blame her. I wouldn't want to get out of that cozy nest while someone else pushed me! I needed to appeal to her Joy Goal to break her out of her comfort zone. It certainly wasn't to run with me, so what could it be?

And like a knight in shining armor, her daddy appeared at the finish and started walking toward us. He wasn't keen on running the 5K either (the things I drag my family to), but he did show up to greet us at the end. Our little girl forgot all about her cold arms and ran toward him. And when she reached him...

She kept running. Okay, so apparently her daddy wasn't the Joy Goal either. Maybe it was the finish line?

She kept running.

By this time I was sprinting too, trying to catch up to her so I wouldn't lose her in the crowd.

Where was she going?

After I cross the finished line, I looked frantically for her. And guess where I found her?

At the pizza table.

The finish line was not the end of the race, but the prize ahead—the pizza! I laughed at how much pull pizza had over this little girl and then thought about how she showed me something profound that day. Our finish line is not simply to make it to the end of life, but to reach the prize of life. We don't exercise to stay healthy so we can die without pain, or boast about having lived a long life with fewer wrinkles than the next person. We run for the joy set before us—the Lord Jesus! And His reward is even better than hot pizza.

> *"...looking to Jesus, the founder*
> *and perfecter of our faith..."*
> HEBREWS 12:2

This chapter is the last leg of our journey together. I want to leave you with permission to change directions with your fitness routine, to take breaks, to count it all joy, and to walk away empowered with the wisdom of the Spirit, knowing what is best for your season. Throughout it all, I want us to stay focused on one person: Jesus. When the shiny objects of life threaten to pull you astray and the myth of more sends you in the wrong direction, keep your eyes on Him. This is how the writer of Hebrews spurred God's people on to endure: "looking to Jesus." He is our long-term maintenance plan. To lay out the long game, let's shine a light on the potholes of distraction and shame, point out the value of being patient in perseverance, and set up a back-up plan for when the storms of life come our way.

1. Isolating the Enemies of Distraction and Shame

"...who for the joy that was set before him endured the cross, despising the shame, and is seated at the right hand of the throne of God."
HEBREWS 12:2

What if Jesus never went to the cross? What if he said it was too hard, or didn't make sense, or gave in to all those who tried to deter him? If Jesus didn't go through with His mission, we would not have the joy of our salvation, the joy that can never be taken away. Nevertheless, the enemy will try and cover our joy under heavy heaps of distraction and shame. He tried the same tricks with Jesus too. But Jesus brushed it all off and stayed the course. How did he stay so free and full of joy? Let's follow His journey.

Despise the Shame

Hebrews 12:2 says Jesus despised the shame. He set it aside and counted it as nothing in comparison to joy set before Him. What is the shame you face in exercise, and how does it affect you? One example is feeling shame over the weight creeping back up, which leads to blaming oneself, which leads to fear of failing again.

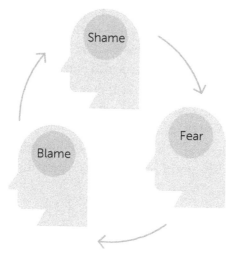

How do we turn this spiral of shame into a circuit of joy? We plug in the loose ends to the joy of the Lord. Linda shares how God broke her out of a shame cycle:

> *God is bringing back my joy for swimming. I quit about five years ago when someone grouched at me at the pool. It wasn't the grouching that made me quit, but the feeling that I didn't belong, didn't deserve to be there. Flash forward with a wrecked knee now, I'm back at swimming to fight for my health. I go to a water aerobics class, and it is so crowded. Yesterday I felt like I was in the way, that I didn't belong there. I thought, 'Maybe I will quit and just swim laps in the future.'*
>
> *While swimming laps after class like usual, I heard from God: 'You are a royal daughter of God, you absolutely have a place at the table; go and claim your place. You are just as deserving to be there as anyone else.' Wow, the joy in that! I'm not going to quit. There is still a lot of healing left around the insecurity of not belonging. But with God's help, I'm on my way!*

Linda felt the **shame** of feeling like she didn't quite belong, and then someone reinforced that feeling by saying something unkind. That made it easier to place the **blame** for not wanting to participate in a crowded class, leading to an increased aversional **fear** of the people there viewing her as an outsider. Jesus was an outsider too. He was crucified outside the city and rejected by His own people. He speaks to her as a friend who has been there, and a King who has overcome. She felt the shame of what others saw, but He reminded her of what He sees: a beloved daughter, chosen, and loved. Once she connected with the truth of the Looker, the joy of His confidence surged through her and moved her to take action.

Name your shame surrounding fitness:

_____

_____

_____

_____

_____

Whom are you blaming, and why?

_____

_____

_____

_____

_____

What do you fear?

_____

_____

_____

_____

_____

Imagine Jesus speaking these words based on your core verse to you, and let His joy move you!

Looker: "You are chosen, holy, and beloved. Step into your royal role." (based on Colossians 3:12)

Freebird: "You are my temple. Meet Me there." (based on 1 Corinthians 6:19)

Hero: "I made you to be filled with My life. I want you to give your life away." (based on 2 Timothy 2:21)

Warrior: "You are a member of My body. I need you to build up others in My love." (based on Ephesians 4:15-16)

Keeper: "You please me. Walk in my approval." (based on 2 Corinthians 5:9)

Re-Member: Distractions and Discouragement

While shame holds us down, distractions throw us off course. When Ephesians 6 says to "take up the shield of faith, with which you can extinguish all the flaming darts of the evil one;" those flaming darts are an old battle tactic used as a diversion. If you're always putting out fires, you miss out on your Joy Goal. A distracted mind disconnects the brain, which responds in one way by releasing the protective stress hormone cortisol to restore homeostasis. We enter into temporary survival mode and look inward, rather than out ahead at our long-distance aim.

Let us remember Jesus on our journey to holistic joy in mind, body, and spirit. To remember is to re-member, to let Him connect our circuits for a whole-body experience. A centered mind bound by joy stabilizes core functions like heart rate and insulin levels. A body at peace has room to stop, pray, and reset focus.

Two main sources of sneaky distraction for our goals are

difficulty and a distorted view of the finish line. When a workout feels too hard, we will avoid it at all costs, forgetting to rely
on the joy of the Lord as our strength. When we forget why we
started, we will get distracted by all the other demands of life.
Let's look at a few of the distractions that try to discourage us,
the same ones that tried to keep Jesus from the cross:

Looker: The Looker is tempted to be swayed and distracted by
popular opinion. Jesus' best friend, Peter, tried to keep Him from
the cross. Your friends and family may not understand why you
make certain sacrifices to work out. Put any accusations behind
you and rise up in who God created you to be. The world needs
you to reflect the light of His joy!

Freebird: You might be distracted by what feels good, perhaps
by lying on the couch and numbing out instead of getting out to
move. Peter, James, and John submitted to sleep in the Garden
of Gethsemane when Jesus needed them most. Who knows what
(or whose) joy could be on the line when you follow the flesh for
satisfaction instead of peace in the Lord's presence?

Hero: The Hero can be distracted by holding back energy in a
workout in an attempt to save her resources. When Mary Mag-
dalene anointed Jesus with expensive perfume, Judas scolded
her for unwise spending. When you exercise, you can find joy
by giving all you have as an outrageous offering to the Lord.
You might find that the more you give, the more joy you'll have!

Warrior: You can be distracted by public displays of victory.
If your team doesn't win or you don't finish a workout, it can
feel like you lost. Jesus' death on the cross looked like defeat.
Everyone deserted him, and he endured alone. You can find joy
knowing that because Jesus has won heaven through humility,
so have you. And He will never leave you. May every workout
be a victory lap celebration with Him!

Keeper: The Keeper is distracted by trying to please others (or earn self value) by adhering to a workout plan instead of listening to the plans of the Lord. Instead of giving a defense to Pilate and the high priest, the ruling authorities of his day, Jesus remained obedient to His Father alone. You can find joy in obeying the Lord in the small things, like holding a plank ten seconds more than you want, or going through a full range of motion instead of doing an exercise half-heartedly. Nobody else may give you credit, but the Lord sees it all, keeps close accounts, and treasures every act of faith.

Focus on the Prize

Even when we get distracted, we can always get back on track by visualizing our Joy Goal as if it is reality. When asked about how she chooses her meals, track and field Olympian Allyson Felix responds, "Nutritious food makes me feel good and perform well. Processed and junk food makes me feel tired and bloated—not a gold medal feeling!"[114] Every decision she makes is for that medal. May every decision we make be for that seasonal Joy Goal. And as our seasons change, may our life-long medal be the joy of the Lord, who has an "inheritance that is imperishable, undefiled, and unfading, kept in heaven for you" (1 Peter 1:4). Just as Felix asks herself throughout each day's choices, "Is this gold medal worthy?" May we ask that of our fitness journey: "Does this decision lead to my Joy Goal?"

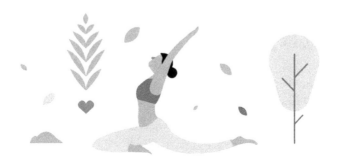

How does looking to Jesus recenter your fitness focus?

_____

_____

_____

_____

_____

2. Persistence and Patience

"Consider him who endured from sinners such hostility against himself, so that you may not grow weary or fainthearted.

In your struggle against sin you have not yet resisted to the point of shedding your blood. And have you forgotten the exhortation that addresses you as sons?

'My son, do not regard lightly the discipline of the Lord, nor be weary when reproved by him.

For the Lord disciplines the one he loves, and chastises every son whom he receives.'

It is for discipline that you have to endure. God is treating you as sons. For what son is there whom his father does not discipline?"

Hebrews 12:3-7

These two words have great power to lift the weight of weari-
ness: "consider Him." When you feel like you can't keep going,
consider Him. When all the effort of keeping up with your own
body seems like too much, consider Him. Consider the hostility
he endured from sinners (including you and me) and how He
pressed on for joy until the end. Then ask Him for strength to
withstand the hostility you face.

> *"Motivation is what gets you started.*
> *Habit is what keeps you going."*
> JIM RYUN[115]

Willpower is not the same as discipline. Willpower is like a
muscle. It fatigues over time. It is strongest in beginning: the
beginning of the day, the week, a new season. This is part of
the reason why Mondays are the most popular days at the gym
and why New Year's resolutions don't last all year. Willpower
is like the first energy system in our body to be used when we
start moving, powered by fast-twitch muscle fibers and great
for sprinting for about thirty seconds—it is a powerful initiator
but short-lived. Discipline is like the aerobic system in our body
that uses oxygen and can be sustained over time—it takes longer
to kick into gear but proves to be longer-lasting. We need both
willpower to start and the habits of discipline to continue.

Self-Discipline is Self-Care

We might not always feel like working out, but the discipline
of habit can condition us for a routine: "the emotional brain
is a follower. You need to use your prefrontal cortex to nudge
it into shape, which means repeatedly rousing it out of its old
way of operating."[116] Repeatedly rousing our emotional brains
to follow along is like parenting. I feel like I'm always herding
my daughter to take care of herself—to get ready for bed, brush
her teeth, and finish her veggies. Eventually, she will do these

things on her own. But even when she reaches adulthood, she still needs a Shepherd.

I realize that self-care these days is defined by treating oneself with bubble baths and chocolate, but self-care is allowing ourselves to be parented. Adults are still sons and daughters. Our Father wants to lead us to the green pastures and quiet waters of joy, but we have to pick up our feet to get there. Walking in discipline is the best self-care. *Thayer's Greek Lexicon* describes *discipline* as "whatever in adults also cultivates the soul, especially by correcting mistakes and curbing the passions."[117]

Michelle's concept of discipline was rooted in school standards, but the Lord wanted to correct her view and cultivate joy:

I realized that I have held onto a belief that moving was something I could do, but also something to be endured, to be obedient in, to be faithful to do. But it was hard, sweaty drudgery that I had no desire to do because I was not good at it. My first experiences with 'physical fitness' were not positive for me as a kid. I did not enjoy gym. I always felt measured, timed, defeated, and last. It wasn't that I was lazy or lethargic; I tried, and I just wasn't good at it. That was hard for this people-pleasing, overachieving heart. So I avoided it... if I couldn't be good, there was no need to pursue it at all. I was talented and acknowledged in other areas. I was friendly, smart, and I could sing. I found my friends in choir, got good grades, and spent my time doing all the things that got me a smile and an atta-girl.

As an adult, if I moved it was because I should, and out of obedience, I would, but not joyfully. All duty, zero enjoyment. But yesterday, Kara, my tribe leader, said three words in the middle of a workout that shifted something deep in me. She said, 'Find your joy' and there was the moment...this unmeasured, untimed, foundation-shifting, powerful freedom moment. Afterwards, I said to myself, 'I almost enjoyed that,' with a smile forming inside. Somewhere within, I heard the Lord whisper, 'It could be like this everyday, just come and move, just me and you.'

What is your idea of discipline?

_____

_____

_____

_____

What is your idea of self-care?

_____

_____

_____

_____

How can moving for joy reconcile the two?

_____

_____

_____

_____

Be Patient

A lifelong habit takes endurance, which means practicing patience. When I watched my daughter try somersaults for the first time at gymnastics, she got impatient. She put her head on the floor, kicked her legs up, but nothing happened. She got up, looked around, stomped her feet, and put her hands up in a frustrated posture with raised eyebrows as if to say, "Why can't I do this?!" I wanted to send her a telekinetic message from across the gym encouraging her: "Be patient with your body! It needs many movements to establish a new motor pattern. You're doing great. Keep your eyes on your teacher, be patient with yourself, and enjoy the process." Lord knows I need to hear those same words for myself: to keep my eyes on the Teacher, receive grace, and have fun.

Through repetition, we train patience, get better, and eventually feel like the movement is an integral part of us:

- *Repetition is the cure for picky movers:* It takes multiple exposures to new foods to develop a taste for it. If I want to start liking broccoli, all the picky eater advice recommends I eat it in many different ways (raw, roasted, smashed, in a soup) and in different environments (at home in a salad, at a restaurant beside a burger, in a park as a snack). The same goes for movement. If there is something you want to learn to enjoy, like running, try running slow, fast, backwards, and in intervals. Try running by yourself in a park, while praying for your neighborhood, on a treadmill with a podcast, or early in the morning with friends. You might surprise yourself with what you become accustomed to, and you may even start to crave it!
- *Repetition makes it easier:* Our first time doing a movement is hard. We don't like being humiliated. The first time I tried snowboarding, I fell flat on my face, skid down an entire hill on my bottom, and had to be wrenched out of a snowpile. But the more I tried, the better I got. The

bunny hill became easy, and I moved on to bigger slopes and more exciting routes. Once we get the autonomy and mastery part down through repetition, it gets easier and we feel ready to move up to the next level.

- *Repetition turns you into a movement prophet:*

"A good hockey player plays where the puck is. A great hockey player plays where the puck is going to be"
Wayne Gretzky

Athletes seem to have an uncanny ability to predict the future of the next play. It's not a superpower or magic move, it's the fruit of patience and practice. The more we train, the stronger our neurological connections respond with more accuracy and speed. When we were born, we waved our hands in front of our faces like foreign objects. But just as we learned to move our hands in sync with our will, so we can learn how to gain greater reign over a skill or sport.

There is one caveat to the benefits of repetition. We like doing things we are good at, but but if we stick to the same activities, our smart bodies will adapt. Doing the same workout for more than three months will cause you to plateau, and you'll wonder why nothing is changing and you'll be frustrated. Our bodies need change in order to change. We need to add stress so our bodies will get stronger to adapt to the new stressor. This concept in fitness terminology is called progressive overload. It doesn't meant you have to completely switch activities, but once you can confidently master a move, it is wise to slowly add in challenges. This can be in the form of adding weight to increase strength, doing single-leg exercises to increase balance, and adding distance to increase endurance.

3. Reminders and a Contingency Plan

Another practical way to stay focused is to continuously surround ourselves with effective reminders that match our prime motivations. These reminders are like rails to the strait and narrow path, where we can safely practice repetition, continuously placing one foot in front of the other, to get to our final destination. Here are a few reminders ordered by the five motivators to help keep you on track to move for joy in the Lord:

Looker: Set up visual reminders
- Take a picture of you moving for joy and save it as your phone background or profile picture. This visual cue will remind you how good exercise makes you feel and how happy you look doing it, sweat and all!
- Write, "I am chosen, holy, and beloved" on your mirrors with dry erase marker.
- Pack your gym bag for the next day, and set it in a high traffic area so you won't miss it.
- Post your work out schedule on your fridge.
- Set a wake-up alarm on your phone, with a prayer like: "Rise up, crown on, get moving."

Freebird: Get centered
- Try this breath whenever you're stressed to restore calm and shift your focus from stress to peace to motivate you to move accordingly. Breathe in through your nostrils to 50 percent of your lung capacity, then another breathe to 80 percent, then a third breath to fill your lungs and expand your diaphragm. Release through a long exhale, feeling a dropping sensation below your navel and pausing at the bottom. Do it during a stress trigger, like being stuck in traffic or in the middle of an argument.
- Feel your feet on the ground. This is where you are, and this is where you start. The Lord is here.

- The five categories of fitness are: Cardiovascular endurance, muscular endurance, muscular strength, flexibility, and body composition.

After de-stressing through breath and body awareness, highlight the areas above you would like to grow in.

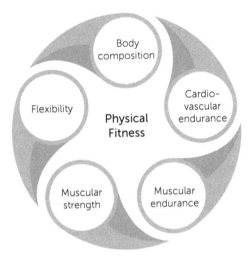

- Add structure: Anchor your loose plans with a schedule. Plan your workouts at the beginning of each week so there are no unknowns, and consider using a paper planner to avoid digital distractions. Pull the areas from above into movements that already bring you joy. For example, if you love to dance and need to add muscular strength, consider adding light hand weights to your pre-planned dance session.

Hero: Focus on filling up
- Find your uninterrupted time: Figure out when you can work out without any interruptions. It could be early in the morning before it's socially appropriate to send email, or at night when everyone is winding down and the kids are asleep.

- Block out your workouts as warm-ups: As you set appointments to take care of business, schedule a workout that will support the business of your day, whether that be a corporate meeting or a parenting play date. Consider your workout as a work warm-up, a non-negotiable schedule block that feeds the rest of your day.
- Celebrate work milestones in your day by taking a movement break. For example, setting a timer to work for forty-five minutes and doing a yoga sequence, or making it to 5 p.m. and having a mini dance party.
- Use timers as boundary lines. Set a timer at the start of your workout so you know exactly how long you have and can fill up the time efficiently.

Warrior: Invite others
- Have a standing weekly workout appointment you can invite others to, like a run outside or class at the gym.
- Check in with your workout buddy on a set weekly time.
- Use operant conditioning by setting up one goal to complete each week, like challenging yourself to add in one exercise session or attempting a higher box jump.
- Grab a friend and sign up for a race together, or sign up alone and find someone else to train with.
- Challenge someone to a steps competition with a fitness tracker. Set the tracker to remind you when you need to get in extra steps.

Keeper: Build reminders into your regular routine
- Wear your workout clothes for pajamas to make getting morning exercise a no-brainer. If you're a parent, just buy athleisure clothes as your wardrobe so you'll be ready to move at all times.
- When getting ready for work, pack yourself a gym bag in addition to a lunch. Keep an extra gym bag in the car in case you forget something.

- During your workouts, set up interval timers with a pleasant ding as a reminder to celebrate short finish lines.
- Install a pull-up bar in a doorway and do one (or a thirty-second hang) every time you pass through.
- Put up an old-fashioned reward chart on your fridge, complete with star stickers.
- Hire a personal trainer to text you reminders to move throughout the week.

Contingency Plan

When (not if) your fitness plan doesn't go according to Plan A, adapt! "Survival of the fittest" means we use fitness to adapt to our circumstances, not adapt our circumstances to our fitness. Too many times, I see people (including myself) give up or fail to start for fear of not being able to master every detail. Wanting to do things right is paralyzing when it comes to worldly challenges. The root of this desire, a hallmark of the Keeper, is a God-given one. We *are* called to be all in. But it's not to an exercise plan. We do not pledge allegiance to a measure of fitness but walk in full faithfulness to the Lord. He wants us to give Him everything we've got! Including our failed plans. If we want to see His true strength in us, we have to give over our weaknesses, our forgetfulness, our injuries, our limited perspective. Our way may not be the only way. So let's open up the possibilities for what He may have in store for us in the form of alternative routes, or backup plans.

The key to a contingency plan is to have the plan set ahead of time. When you're in emergency mode, it's harder to think of an alternative, and often a workout just won't happen. If you planned to go to the gym, but sleep in, have a window of time ready during the day that you can fit in fitness, such as swapping downtime right before dinner to do twenty minutes of an at-home workout. When you have planned to do cardio outdoors but it's storming outside, have another routine in your wheelhouse you can do indoors. This can include creating a YouTube cardio playlist ahead of time, or memorizing a high intensity bodyweight interval series like the one below.

Sample indoor cardio series: thirty seconds each of mountain climbers, skaters, burpees, and high knees as fast as you can. Rest one minute and repeat for three rounds. Swap out exercises as needed. For a simple strength set, try 25 push-ups, 25 squats, a 1-minute plank, and a 1-minute superman hold. Repeat for four sets.

What is your contingency plan? In the first row, write out your ideal workout week from Chapter Nine, and in the second row, write a Plan B.

SUN	Ideal workout	
	Plan B	
MON	Ideal workout	
	Plan B	
TUES	Ideal workout	
	Plan B	
WED	Ideal workout	
	Plan B	

THU	Ideal workout	
	Plan B	
FRI	Ideal workout	
	Plan B	
SAT	Ideal workout	
	Plan B	

I could have written this book in one sentence: "Move for joy: just do it and you'll see!" But that wouldn't have been nearly as much fun as writing a whole book, just as an endorphin-infused pill wouldn't be as rewarding as exercise. Even when we don't want to, we can still move our bodies, let our hearts catch up, and complete the circuit of joy:

> In response to 'not feeling like it' "the biblical response to that is, 'Lift up your praising hands to the Holy Place, and bless God!' You can lift up your hands regardless of how you feel; it is a simple motor movement. You may not be able to command your heart, but you can command your arms. Lift your arms in blessing; just maybe your heart will get the message and also be lifted up in praise. We are psychosomatic beings; body and spirit are intricately inter-related. Go through the motions of blessing God, and your spirit will pick up the cue and follow along. 'For why do men lift their hands when they pray? Is it not that their hearts may be raised at the same time to God?'[118]

Exercise:

My daughter likes to be independent. She loves growing in autonomy, so I let her practice mastery (and let her fail to learn from her mistakes, too). She will get her own cup and fill it up with water—all the way to the brim. For kids, if the glass isn't full, it's empty. She looks down at her cup and moves toward the table at snail speed, sloshing water all over the place. I make a suggestion to her: "Look at the table, not at your cup" (maybe I should have put pizza on the table and she would move faster). She listened. She moved more gracefully and didn't spill any more water.

This is the same concept as a balance beam. The closer you look at your feet as you move, the more off balance you will become. Try walking heel-to-toe while looking straight down at your feet. Now try it while looking ahead to the end of your route. Let this be a reminder that when your fitness journey is hard to navigate, listen to the Lord, lift your head, and focus on the joy of Jesus set before you and within you. He is with us in the journey, and there at the finish line.

Invitation to More

Dearest reader,

Thank you for walking on the joy journey with me! I realize that fitness is only one part of the equation of our health and fitness journey. If you are interested in individual faith-based health coaching with group accountability with more of a nutrition component, learn more about our services at *kaseybshuler.com/shop/moveforjoy*.

We realize that sometimes you need a real person to help you identify personal goals, obstacles, and practical next steps. Here's how just the fitness coaching portion has helped others:

"I'm not a real goal-setter or reverse-engineer person. I think 'I'll just wing it!' I don't come up with specific outcomes. But figuring out at the start of my week how I want to feel by the end is key. It totally makes sense to me. Having the opportunity to externally process and talk it out and, having the time to think about why I do what I do and where to go next has been so helpful." -Jessica

"Part of my personality is that I don't share a lot of my own goals. Having the opportunity to go over the things I want to do and accomplish was good." -Andrew

"Anytime I write things down, I'm more likely to reach my goals. It's helpful to focus and verbalize it all. I appreciate taking the fitness aspect and centering it around the Lord. It's easy to focus on the external benefits, like trying to lose

baby weight, but this helps me remember that God gave me this body, which makes others." -Emily

I want to continue this journey with you. If you do nothing else, sign up for my email list at **kaseybshuler.com** so we can stay connected. I hope to meet and work with you soon.

For joy,
Kasey Shuler

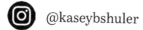 @kaseybshuler

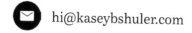 hi@kaseybshuler.com

Bonus Chapter

Quick Ways to Spark Joy

The weekend started with a gymnasium full of 200 women ready to work out, ready to receive a blessing at Rev on the Road for Revelation Wellness. We were all freezing, wrapped in sweatshirts when we showed up that morning. When it was time for lunch, our bodies were not only sweating, but the room was significantly warmer. We didn't turn up the heat on the thermostat, we turned up the heat by drumming to the beat, jacking in sync, and flowing into poses with precision. The magnitude of that moment struck me: we are the light of the world! We shine by showing up, and we produce warmth by moving.

If showing up is half the battle, then getting past the warm-up is the other half. The warm-up is the initial transition period of your body to break through the barrier from resting to cardio. It doesn't matter how long you've been exercising; this part is always hard. Warming up literally increases your body temperature a few degrees. The happy neurochemicals start to kick in around minute seven or eight, so think less about doing an hour-long workout and more about an eight-minute workout. Once you get past the warm-up, you'll be on fire and want to keep it burning. Your body even has its own built-in sprinkler system: sweat! God really did think of everything.

But sometimes, we simply need a spark of joy to get the fire going and get us moving. When is the last time you played without performing? When is the last time you laughed, I mean really laughed? If you can't recall, you're not alone:

> *"I enjoy being creative—drawing, coloring, painting, making music… last time I belly laughed? I think I was watching the video of the lady with the Chewbacca mask. I need to spend more time doing all those things that I enjoy doing, plus spend more time outside, to increase joy in my life." -Elizabeth*

> *"I'm praying for grace, courage, clarity, and for the power of God to do what I cannot. I continually surrender and remain eating how I feel God wants me to. Yet I see little change. I pray He brings this joy back into my life. Meanwhile I trust in His love and His promises." -Jodee*

> *"How often I try to conjure up my own joy and happiness. I am learning to press into the Lord so it is HIS joy that becomes my strength." -Ronda*

When you have lost or forgotten your joy, link arms with these women—pray, continue being obedient, and wait on the Lord. I may have a few activities in mind for you while you're waiting. When your original plan goes awry and you need a quick backup option, or simply need quick reference point to spark your joy, check out the list below and get that fire going. The following ideas are categorized by mood, to remedy a feeling; or mode, to work with a situation you're in.

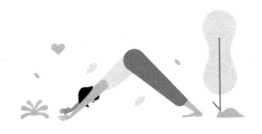

MOOD

When you're tired and grumpy:

"Dancing helps me shake off the funk." -Laura

- Bounce your shoulders up and down
- Turn on the hokey pokey and follow the instructions
- Move your arms in place as fast as you can, imagining yourself running at breakneck speed
- Jump in a cold body of water
- Go outside and race a squirrel
- Try to catch falling leaves

When you're stressed and need to be with people:

"Usually a good hike with a friend, a walk with my dog, or outdoor activity makes me feel most alive. Nature is calming and somehow reflective for me. I believe God speaks to me often in those moments." -Michelle

- Message your neighbor or a friend to go on a walk
- Head to a fitness studio or gym (especially for a class)
- Peruse apps to find fitness friends like Fitness Buddy or Workout Buddies
- When none of your friends can join you, go to a populated park, and walk around just to be around people. And the more often you go at the same time, the more likely you are to gain a fitness friend!

When you're overwhelmed and need to get away:

"I was very depressed and began running and it healed my body! I have a wonderful friendship with running!" -Luan

- Close your eyes and do a stretching sequence

- Go out to a safe, public spot on the outskirts of town or on a trail
- Drive out to a favorite hiking spot

When you're bored:

"I always say that feeling the cold on my skin makes me feel alive. Something about the cold and wind remind me of my smallness and therefore make me feel alive." -Joy

- Challenge yourself
  - See how many repetitions of a safe bodyweight exercise you can do in one minute
  - Throw a medicine ball as far as you can, and try to grab it before it stops rolling
  - Throw a ball up high, and see how many jumping jacks you can do before catching it
- Swing as high as you can at a playground
- Go to a local salsa lesson or line dancing class
- Make your own obstacle course
- Call a friend to play tennis, basketball, frisbee, or other sport of choice
- Sign up for a different workout studio in town
- Challenge a friend on a fitness app

When you don't want to exercise, but do want to catch up on media:

"What makes me feel alive? The energy I get after a good run listening to worship music." -Jamie

- Put in your headphones and listen to a podcast, audible book, or playlist
- Take your favorite show mobile and find a recumbent bike, or challenge yourself to keep your upper body stable on

another cardio machine so you don't bounce all around trying to watch
- While reading a book: walk around, do side leg lifts, squats, planks, or anything else that can keep your body moving and your mind focused on the pages

When you're lacking inspiration:

"When I run or bike, I can just move with the Lord's guidance and I'm not counting or predicting the next tempo change. There's less of me when I run or bike, and therefore, there is more of Him in that movement. So I can hear Him loud and clear and I'm not talking over Him." -Linda

- Do a repetitive exercise like walking, swimming, or biking to shut down your worry centers and open up creative space
- Simulate a think tank by going to the pool and spending some time underwater
- Do cross-body, side-to-side movements to integrate your brain hemispheres
- Go on a walk and call a friend, or invite someone to go with you to verbalize your thoughts
- Travel to a scenic spot and explore nature

When you could use a spontaneous adventure, go:

- Rock climbing
- Paddle boarding (SUP yoga)
- Parkour
- Aerial yoga
- Set up a local walking scavenger hunt

MODE

When you're stuck with kids at home:

- 5-minute freeze dance parties: Curate a fun family-friendly playlist for impromptu shenanigans
- Outside walks: carry kids on your back, race them, engage them in tag
- If it's fall, try to catch the falling leaves. If it's snowing, build a snowman. If it's summer, run through the sprinklers.
- Kid-friendly YouTube workouts: Cosmic Kids Yoga, Revelation Wellness, REFITREV dance videos, Go Noodle
- Video game fitness

When you have to work overtime:

- Drink more water to cause more walking via bathroom breaks
- Visit desks instead of sending emails
- Park farther away
- Take stairs instead of elevator
- Set an alarm every hour, to do stretching sequence
- Walking meetings
- Find a good spot for a picnic lunch, and walk around the building afterwards to aid digestion

When you don't have time aside from your routine:

- Pretend you have no car, and do more urban hiking
- Pretend you have no furniture, which forces you to sit all the way on the ground and back up
- Take on a weekend home or outdoor improvement project
- Engage in speed errands
- Take lunch hour walk breaks

- Do more household tasks
- Get outside to garden
- Progress activities of daily living: try and make a movement lower, higher, longer, or go faster or harder

Acknowledgements

"Ack! The Acknowledgements!" is what I said when I finished writing this book. I feel like these people have been with me the whole time, so it feels like an embarrassing oversight that I almost forgot this section. What these people really need is not a shout out, but a huge hug and a big party in their honor. I'm going to get started on planning that. But for now, I'll say it here. This could not have happened without you. Thank you.

Before I start, to anyone who is offended by the order in which you were named, the last will be first. So I'm actually giving you a head start in heaven.

To Mattox, my husband. Five years ago when I whined and moaned about how I had written a book that people couldn't connect with, I mentioned how what we really needed in fitness was not more exercise but more grace. You said, "Now *that* is your book." Your opinions are golden. I treasure them up. Thank you for working late nights with me and encouraging me when I wanted to quit. And for allowing me to write about you.

To Ellie, my daughter. I learn so much from you. I can't wait until you can read this book and know how much you have influenced me to move for joy.

To Mom, the original personal trainer. To Dad, whose lifetime of exercise inspires me. To my sister—who is always up for a good ole Ab Ripper X session.

To Alisa Keeton and the whole Revelation Wellness family: connecting with like-minded brothers and sisters who preach the gospel through fitness completes my joy. Keep delivering the pizza!

To my editor, Danielle. You were with me from the beginning of my health blogging days. This book is what the blog was meant to become. Thank you for making sense out of my ramblings.

To all those who have been unashamed to share their testimonies throughout this book, thank you. Your story for His glory!

To all my clients, past, present, and future. Thank you for respecting your bodies and the Lord enough to hire and inspire me! Your joy is mine.

Notes

1 Augustine, *Confessions*, trans. R.S. Pine-Coffin (New York: Penguin, 1961), 228.

2 "No leisure-time physical activity, adults, 2012," Healthypeople.gov, Office of Disease Prevention and Health Promotion, August 25, 2014, accessed May 23, 2019,

https://www.healthypeople.gov/2020/topics-objectives/national-snapshot/no-leisure-time-physical-activity-adults-2012.

3 Emily Sohn, "Exercise is fundamental to good health. So why do few Americans stick with it?" *The Washington Post*, May 7, 2017, accessed May 23, 2019, https://www.washingtonpost.com/national/health-science/exercise-is-fundamental-to-good-health-so-why-do-few-americans-stick-with-it/2017/05/05/2c537338-2e81-11e7-8674-437ddb6e813e_story.html?noredirect=on&utm_term=.38a7de1c129f.

4 Gretchen Reynolds, *The First 20 Minutes: Surprising Science Reveals How We Can: Exercise Better, Train Smarter, Live Longer* (Hudson Street Press, 2012), 3.

5 Neville Owen, PhD, et al., "Sedentary Behavior: Emerging Evidence for a New Health Risk," *Mayo Clinic Proceedings* 85, no. 12, (December 2010): 1138-1141, https://www.ncbi.nlm.nih.gov/pmc/articles/PMC2996155/.

6 John Naish, "It's not just true about diets, YO-YO EXERCISE makes you fat: Experts reveal resolution-fuelled workout frenzies do not make us fitter," *Daily Mail*, January 9, 2017, accessed May 23, 2019, http://www.dailymail.co.uk/health/article-4103126/It-s-not-just-true-diets-yo-yo-EXERCISE-makes-fat-Experts-reveal-resolution-fuelled-workout-frenzies-not-make-fitter.html.

7 Louise Chang, MD, "Top 6 Exercise Excuses and How to Beat Them," WebMD, April 11, 2012, accessed May 23, 2019, https://www.webmd.com/fitness-exercise/features/the-top-6-exercise-excuses-and-how-to-beat-them#2.

8 *The American Heritage Stedman's Medical Dictionary*, s.v."fitness," accessed May 17, 2019, http://www.dictionary.com/browse/fitness.

9 Mandy Oaklander and Heather Jones, "7 Surprising Benefits of Exercise," *Time*, September 1, 2016, accessed May 23, 2019, http://time.com/4474874/exercise-fitness-workouts/.

10 Lizette Borreli, "Sweat It Out! 5 Surprising Health Benefits of Sweating That Actually Don't Stink," Medical Daily, November 7, 2014, accessed May 23, 2019, https://www.medicaldaily.com/sweat-it-out-5-surprising-health-benefits-sweating-actually-dont-stink-309718.

11 Kathleen M. Hutchinson, Helaine Alessio, and Rachael R. Baiduc, "Association Between Cardiovascular Health and Hearing Function: Pure-Tone and Distortion Product Otoacoustic Emission Measures," *American Journal of Audiology*, (June 1, 2010), https://aja.pubs.asha.org/article.aspx?articleid=1757453.

12 Katy Bowman, "Movement is a Solution," Nutritious Movement, accessed May 18, 2019, https://nutritiousmovement.com/about/.

13 Benjamin Baddeley, Sangeetha Sornalingam, and Max Cooper, "Sitting is the new smoking: where do we stand?" *British Journal of General Practice*, 66, no. 646, (May 2016): 258, https://www.ncbi.nlm.nih.gov/pmc/articles/PMC4838429/.

14 "2018 Physical Activity Guidelines Advisory Committee Scientific Report," Health.gov, accessed May 18, 2019, https://health.gov/paguidelines/second-edition/report/pdf/08_F-2_Sedentary_Behavior.pdf.

15 Erin Hoare, et al., "The associations between sedentary behaviour and mental health among adolescents: a systematic review," *International Journal of Behavioral Nutrition and Physical Activity*, 13, no. 108 (September 2016), https://ijbnpa.biomedcentral.com/articles/10.1186/s12966-016-0432-4.

16 John Ratey, MD, *Spark: The Revolutionary New Science of Exercise and the Brain* (New York: Hatchette Book Group, 2008), 114.

17 "Who do/did you work out at your gym?" Statista, accessed May 18, 2019, https://www.statista.com/statistics/639169/reasons-behind-gym-exercise-in-us/

18 Arabella Ogilvie, "How Much Do Americans Spend On Health and Fitness?" My Protein, accessed May 18, 2019, https://us.myprotein.com/thezone/training/much-americans-spend-health-fitness-survey-results-revealed/.

19 Manda Mahoney, "The Subconscious Mind of the Consumer," Harvard Business School, January 13, 2013, accessed May 23, 2019, https://hbswk.hbs.edu/item/the-subconscious-mind-of-the-consumer-and-how-to-reach-it.

20 Richard Foster, *Celebration of Discipline: The Path to Spiritual Growth*, (New York: Harper Collins, 1998), 108.

21 A.W. Tozer, *Who Put Jesus on the Cross?: And Other Questions of the Christian Faith*, (Chicago: Moody Publishers, 2009), 170.

22 Josh. 6:2, ESV

23 Christopher Bergland, "The Neurochemicals of Happiness," Psychology Today, November 29, 2012, accessed May 23, 2019, https://www.psychologytoday.com/us/blog/the-athletes-way/201211/the-neurochemicals-happiness.

24 Wayne Celeban, "Six Stages of disease - Samprapti," Yukti Botanicals, 2017, accessed May 23, 2019, http://www.yukti.com.au/pages/six-stages-of-disease-samprapti.

25 Judith Orloff MD, "The Health Benefits of Tears," Psychology Today, July 27, 2010, accessed May 23, 2019, https://www.psychologytoday.com/us/blog/emotional-freedom/201007/the-health-benefits-tears.

26 Michelle Segar, PhD, *No Sweat: How the Simple Science of Motivation Can Bring You a Lifetime of Fitness*, (New York: American Management Association, 2015), 6.

27 Steven Pressfield, *The War of Art*, (New York: Black Irish Entertainment LLC, 2002), 1.

28 David Zahl, "What the Heart Loves, the Will Chooses and the Mind Justifies: Ashley Null on Thomas Cranmer," Mockingbird, January 5, 2011, accessed May 23, 2019, http://www.mbird.com/2011/01/ashley-null-via-thomas-cranmer-on/.

29 Larissa Mercado-Lopez, "Who Gets To Be Fit: Working Out the Intersections of Fitness," Girls Gone Strong (blog), March 2016, accessed May 23, 2019, https://www.girlsgonestrong.com/blog/feminism/intersectionality-of-fitness/.

30 K. Ball, D. Crawford, and N. Owen, "Too fat to exercise? Obesity as a barrier to physical activity," *PubMed.gov*, (June 2000), https://www.ncbi.nlm.nih.gov/pubmed/10937415.

31 Natalie Joffe, "5 Strategies to Cultivate Body Respect in a Thin-Privileged World," Girls Gone Strong (blog), May 2018, accessed May 23, 2019 https://www.girlsgonestrong.com/blog/confidence/body-embracement/5-strategies-to-cultivate-body-respect-in-a-thin-privileged-world/?utm_source=6.3.18-community-newsletter&utm_medium=email&utm_campaign=community-newsletter&utm_content=5-strategies-to-cultivate-body-respect-in-a-thin-privileged-world.

32 Titus 2:10b, Berean Study Bible

33 G.K. Chesterton, *Orthodoxy*, (London: William Clowes and Sons, 1934), 21

34 Daniel Amen, *Change Your Brain, Change Your Body: Use Your Brain to Get and Keep the Body You Have Always Wanted*, (New York: Three Rivers Press, 2010).

35 N.T. Wright, *Surprised by Hope: Rethinking Heaven, the Resurrection, and the Mission of the Church*, (New York: HarperOne, 2008).

36 Thomas Cash and Linda Smolak, B*ody Image: A Handbook of Science, Practice, and Prevention*, (New York: The Guilford Press, 2011).

37 Heb. 12:1-3, The Message

38 Daniel Siegel and Tina Bryson, *The Whole-Brain Child: 12 Revolutionary Strategies to Nurture Your Child's Developing Mind*, (New York: Bantam Books, 2012), 61.

39 Craig Williamson, *Muscular Retraining for Pain-Free Living: A Practical Approach to Eliminating Chronic Back Pain, Tendonitis, Neck and Shoulder Tension, and Repetitive Stress Injuries*, (Boston: Trumpeter Books, 2007), 22.

40 John Ratey, MD, *Spark: The Revolutionary New Science of Exercise and the Brain* (New York: Hatchette Book Group, 2008), 101.

41 Gaétan Chevalier, et al., "Earthing: Health Implications of Reconnecting the Human Body to the Earth's Surface Electrons," *Journal of Environmental Public Health*, (January 12, 2012), https://www.ncbi.nlm.nih.gov/pmc/articles/PMC3265077/.

42 Bessel Van Der Kolk, MD, *The Body Keeps The Score: Brain, Mind, and Body In The Healing of Trauma*, (New York: Penguin Books, 2015), 216.

43 Craig Williamson, *Muscular Retraining for Pain-Free Living: A Practical Approach to Eliminating Chronic Back Pain, Tendonitis, Neck and Shoulder Tension, and Repetitive Stress Injuries*, (Boston: Trumpeter Books, 2007), 15.

44 Ps. 16:6

45 "Resources," National Coalition Against Domestic Violence, accessed May 19, 2019, https://ncadv.org/resources.

46 Gregory Bratman, et al., "The Benefits of Nature Experience: Improved Affect and Cognition," *Landscape and Urban Planning*, vol. 138 (June 2015): 41-50, http://www.sciencedirect.com/science/article/pii/S0169204615000286.

47 Rob Jordan, "Stanford Researchers Find Mental Health Prescription: Nature." Stanford, June 30, 2015, accessed May 19, 2019, http://news.stanford.edu/2015/06/30/hiking-mental-health-063015/.

48 James Cowan, *The Effects of Sound on People*, (United Kingdom: John Wiley & Sons, 2016).

49 Q. Li, et al., "Effect of Phytoncide from Trees on Human Natural Killer Cell Function," *PubMed.gov*, (October 2009), https://www.ncbi.nlm.nih.gov/pubmed/20074458/.

50 Richard Foster, *Celebration of Discipline: The Path to Spiritual Growth*, (New York: Harper Collins, 1998), 169.

51 Andrew Newberg and Mark Robert Waldman, *How God Changes Your Brain: Breakthrough Findings from a Leading Neuroscientist*, (New York: Ballantine Books Trade Paperbacks, 2010).

52 Philip Yaffe, "The 7% Rule: Fact, Fiction, or Misunderstanding," *Ubiquity*, vol. 2011 (October 2011): 1-5, https://ubiquity.acm.org/article.cfm?id=2043156..

53 Anne Harding, "Study: Obese Workers, Smokers Less Productive," Health. com, December 10, 2018, accessed May 23, 2019, https://www.health.com/home/ obesity-smoking-productivity.

54 "Exercise during pregnancy is good for mother, baby, research confirms," Plataforma SINC, September 2017, accessed May 23, 2019, https://www.sciencedaily.com/ releases/2017/09/170904093621.htm.

55 "Babies born big more likely to become obese as children, study finds," University of Virginia Health System, July 12, 2017, accessed May 23, 2019, https://www.sciencedaily. com/releases/2017/07/170712110518.htm.

56 Daniel Amen, Change Your Brain, *Change Your Body: Use Your Brain to Get and Keep the Body You Have Always Wanted*, (New York: Three Rivers Press, 2010).

57 Robert Davis, "Better hearing, less constipation, and other surprising benefits of exercise," CNN, March 15, 2018, accessed May 23, 2019, https://www.cnn.com/2017/08/09/health/ hearing-sleep-colds-fitness-exercise-davis/index.html.

58 Katy Bowman, *Movement Matters: Essays on Movement Science, Movement Ecology, and the Nature of Movement*, (Sequiem: Propriometrics Press, 2016).

59 R. Glaser, "Education and Thinking: The Role of Knowledge," Technical Report No. PDS-6, (Pittsburgh, PA: University of Pittsburgh, Learning and Development Center, June 1983).

60 Socrates, *Xenophon*, accessed May 19, 2019, http://perseus.uchicago.edu/perseus-cgi/ citequery3.pl?dbname=GreekFeb2011&getid=1&query=Xen.%20Mem.%203.12.

61 Eccles. 4:4, NIV

62 Brock Armstrong, "The Future of Fitness: Massively Multiplayer Online Training," Quick and Dirty Tips (blog), June 6, 2018, accessed May 23, 2019, https://www.quickanddirtytips. com/health-fitness/exercise/the-future-of-fitness-massively-multiplayer-online-training.

63 Antonia F. de C. Hamilton and Frida Lind, "Audience effects: what can they tell us about social neuroscience, theory of mind and autism?" *Cult Brain*, (October 13, 2016): 159-177, https://www.ncbi.nlm.nih.gov/pmc/articles/PMC5095155/.

64 Vivek Murthy, "Work and the Loneliness Epidemic," *Harvard Business Review*, accessed March 23, 2019, https://hbr.org/cover-story/2017/09/work-and-the-loneliness-epidemic.

65 R.R. Wing and R.W. Jeffery, "Benefits of recruiting participants with friends and increasing social support for weight loss and maintenance," J Consult Clinical Psychology, 67, (February 1999): 132, https://www.ncbi.nlm.nih.gov/pubmed/10028217.

66 Stephanie Paulsell, *Honoring the Body: Meditations on a Christian Practice*, (San Francisco: Jossey-Bass, 2002), 120.

67 "Alétheuó," Strong's Concordance, accessed May 19, 2019, https://biblehub.com/ greek/226.htm.

68 2 Cor. 12:9

69 David Epstein, "Are athletes really getting faster, better, stronger?" TED2014, accessed May 21, 2019, https://www.ted.com/talks/ david_epstein_are_athletes_really_getting_faster_better_stronger/transcript.

70 Brett Stetka, "Have We Reached the Athletic Limits of the Human Body?" *Scientific American*, August 5, 2016, accessed May 23, 2019, https://www.scientificamerican.com/article/have-we-reached-the-athletic-limits-of-the-human-body/.

71 Craig Williamson, *Muscular Retraining for Pain-Free Living: A Practical Approach to Eliminating Chronic Back Pain, Tendonitis, Neck and Shoulder Tension, and Repetitive Stress Injuries*, (Boston: Trumpeter Books, 2007), 15

72 N. Burke, "Group Individual Approach," University of Birmingham, accessed January 2019, http://eprints.bham.ac.uk/426/1/BurkeNtoumanisGroupIndividualApproach.pdf.

73 Deborah Feltz, Norbert Kerr, and Brandon Irwin. "Buddy Up: the Kohler Effect Applied to Health Games," *Journal of Sport & Exercise Psychology*, 33, no. 4, (August 2011): 506-26, https://www.researchgate.net/publication/51539278_Buddy_Up_The_Kohler_Effect_Applied_to_Health_Games.

74 M.W. Kraus, C. Huang, and D. Keltner, "Tactile communication, cooperation, and performance: an ethological study of the NBA," *Emotion*, 10, no. 5 (October 2010): 745-9, https://www.ncbi.nlm.nih.gov/pubmed/21038960.

75 Revelation Wellness - Healthy & Whole. 2017. "Love God. Get Healthy. Be Whole. Love Others," accessed May 23, 2019, https://www.facebook.com/revelationwell/videos/1267208493345178/.

76 John Koessler, *The Radical Pursuit of Rest*, (Downers Grove: InterVarsity Press, 2016).

77 "Active Living," Surgeon General,. U.S. Department of Health & Human Services, accessed November 27, 2016, http://www.surgeongeneral.gov/priorities/prevention/strategy/active-living.html.

78 William Sears and Martha Sears, *The Healthy Pregnancy Book: Month by Month, Everything You Need to Know from America's Baby Experts*, (New York: Little, Brown and Company, 2013), 14.

79 Mandy Oaklander and Heather Jones, "7 Surprising Benefits of Exercise," *Time*, September 1, 2016, accessed May 23, 2019, http://time.com/4474874/exercise-fitness-workouts/.

80 Gretchen Reynolds, *The First 20 Minutes: Surprising Science Reveals How We Can: Exercise Better, Train Smarter, Live Longer* (Hudson Street Press, 2012), 9.

81 Chalene Johnson, "6 Morning Habits For Weight Loss," podcast with Shawn Stevenson, accessed December 2018, https://www.chalenejohnson.com/podcasts/morning-habit-for-weight-loss/.

82 "Anti-Aging Market Report 2018 with Forecasts to 2023," PRNewswire, March 6, 2018, accessed May 23, 2019, https://www.prnewswire.com/news-releases/anti-aging-market-report-2018-with-forecasts-to-2023-300608930.html.

83 Craig Williamson, *Muscular Retraining for Pain-Free Living: A Practical Approach to Eliminating Chronic Back Pain, Tendonitis, Neck and Shoulder Tension, and Repetitive Stress Injuries*, (Boston: Trumpeter Books, 2007), 125.

84 "World's Oldest Person Marks 120 Beautiful, Happy Years," *The Deseret News*, February 21, 1995, accessed May 23, 2019, https://news.google.com/newspapers?id=CL4RAAAAIBAJ&sjid=jOwDAAAAIBAJ&pg=1584,3192209&hl=en.

85 Tara Parker-Pope, "The Surprising Shortcut to Better Health," *The New York Times*, May 4, 2012, accessed May 23, 2019,https://well.blogs.nytimes.com/2012/05/04/the-surprising-shortcut-to-better-health.

86 Dan Buettner, "Power 9," Blue Zones, accessed May 21, 2019, https://www.bluezones.com/2016/11/power-9/.

87 Sam Wong, "Walking to work cuts risk of diabetes and high blood pressure," Imperial College London, August 6, 2013, https://www.imperial.ac.uk/news/127087/walking-work-cuts-risk-diabetes-high/.

88 Alisa Keeton, "People often ask me how much I workout," Instagram, July 18, 2018, accessed May 23, 2019, https://www.instagram.com/p/BlYju1_AQXT/?taken-by=alisakeeton.

89 Anne Lamott, *Small Victories: Spotting Imporbably Moments of Grace*, (New York: Riverhead Books, 2014),159.

90 "Philotimeomai," Strong's Concordance, accessed May 21, 2019, https://biblehub.com/greek/5389.htm.

91 Dan Buettner, *The Blue Zones, Second Edition: 9 Lessons for Living Longer From the People Who've Lived the Longest*, (Washington, D.C.: The National Geographic Society, 2012).

92 John 21:15

93 Richard Foster, *Celebration of Discipline: The Path to Spiritual Growth*, (New York: Harper Collins, 1998), 80.

94 "Hebrews 12," Ellicott's Commentary for English Readers, accessed May 21, 2019, https://biblehub.com/commentaries/ellicott/hebrews/12.htm.

95 "ACE Integrated Fitness Training Model," ACE, accessed May 21, 2019, https://www.acefitness.org/fitness-certifications/personal-trainer-certification/ace-ift-model.aspx.

96 Alice Park, "How Exercise Keeps Your DNA Young," July 27, 2016, accessed May 23, 2019, http://time.com/4426572/exercise-dna-telomeres/?iid=sr-link2.

97 C.S. Lewis, *Problem of Pain*, (New York: Harper Collins, 1996).

98 Aubrey Golbek, *Grace, Food, and Everything in Between: Discover the Transforming Power of Grace to Set You Free From Food and Body Shame*, (Amazon, 2018).

99 Bonnie Berkowitz, Shelly Tan, and Seth Blanchard, "Which Olympic Sports Fit Your Body?" *The Washington Post*, August 10, 2016, accessed May 23, 2019, https://www.washingtonpost.com/graphics/sports/olympics/olympic-body-types/?noredirect=on.

100 Boris Gutnik, et al., "Body physique and dominant somatotype in elite and low-profile athletes with different specializations," Medicina, 51, no. 4, (2015): 247-252, https://www.sciencedirect.com/science/article/pii/S1010660X15000518.

101 John Calvin, *The Institutes of the Christian Religion*, trans. Henry Beveridge (Edinburgh: Calvin Translation Society, 1846), accessed May 22, 2019, https://oll.libertyfund.org/titles/535.

102 A.L. Hicks, J. Kent-Braun, and D.S. Ditor, "Sex differences in human skeletal muscle fatigue." *Exercise and Sports Sciences Review* 29, no. 3, (2001) 109–112.

103 R.H. Fitts and J.J. Widrick, "Muscle mechanics: adaptations with exercise-training," *Exercise and Sport Sciences Reviews* 24, (1996) 0091-6331.

104 Liz Plosser, *Women's Health Magazine*, June 2018, 112.

105 Ronan Leonard, "Habits Maketh the Man," Medium (blog), December 13, 2016, accessed May 23, 2019, https://medium.com/swlh/habits-maketh-the-man-32fd07037a6.

106 Christopher Bergland, *The Athlete's Way*, (New York: St. Martin's Press, 2007).

107 Melia Robinson, "What 'Unbreakable Kimmy Schmidt' taught me about the power of mantras," Tech Insider, March 14, 2016, accessed May 26, 2019, https://www.businessinsider.com/unbreakable-kimmy-schmidt-ten-seconds-mantra-2016-3.

108 "2008 Physical Guidelines for Americans Summary," health.gov, accessed May 23, 2019, https://health.gov/paguidelines/guidelines/summary.aspx.

109 Daniel Plink, *Drive: The Surprising Truth About What Motivates Us*, (New York: Riverhead Press, 2009), 217.

110 Eugene Peterson, *A Long Obedience in the Same Direction: Discipleship in an Instant Society*, (Downers Grove:Intervarsity Press, 2000), 99.

111 Scott Sonnon, "Intuitive Training Defined!" Bodybuilding, January 22, 2019, accessed May 27, 2019, https://www.bodybuilding.com/fun/sonnon4.htm.

112 Eugene Peterson, *A Long Obedience in the Same Direction: Discipleship in an Instant Society*, (Downers Grove:Intervarsity Press, 2000).

113 "Standing Long Jump Test (Broad Jump)," Topend Sports, accessed May 21, 2019, https://www.topendsports.com/testing/tests/longjump.htm.

114 Julie Mazziotta, Julie, "Olympian Allyson Felix's Food Diary: What I Eat in a Day," PEOPLE.com, July 14, 2016, accessed May 23, 2019. http://people.com/food/allyson-felix-food-diary/.

115 Jessica Wei, "Motivation is What Gets You Started," Due, January 16, 2016, accessed May 29, 2019, https://due.com/blog/motivation-gets-started-jim-ryun/.

116 Laurel Mellin, *Wired for Joy!: A Revolutionary Method for Creating Happiness Within*, (Carlsbad, Hay House Inc., 2010), 132.

117 "Paideia," Strong's Concordance, accessed May 21, 2019, https://biblehub.com/greek/3809.htm.

118 Eugene Peterson, *A Long Obedience in the Same Direction: Discipleship in an Instant Society*, (Downers Grove:Intervarsity Press, 2000), 194.

Other resources from Kasey

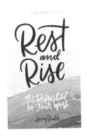

Rest and Rise

Discover the powerful practice of rest as this 4-week study guides you through real ways to answer Jesus's invitation in Matthew 11:28-30. You will develop a daily rhythm of solitude in God's presence as you dive deep into the biblical blessings of rest.

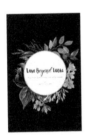

Love Beyond Looks

Your body changes, but God's love for you will not! In this 5-week study, you'll discover how God sees you and loves you as you are through the mirror of His Word.

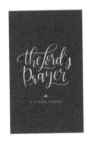

The Lord's Prayer: A 12-Week Journal

Not sure how to pray? This journal breaks down the Lord's prayer into morning and evening templates for a week, starting with the a Sabbath day and ending with free-writing pages. Including prompts to pray for each group of people in your life, this journal will help give you focus in the way Jesus taught us to pray.

Learn more at kaseybshuler.com/shop

CPSIA information can be obtained
at www.ICGtesting.com
Printed in the USA
LVHW081625280420
654675LV00019B/2137